organic
LIVING

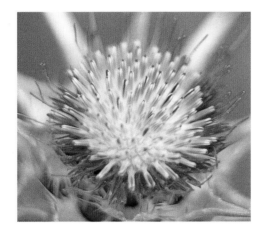

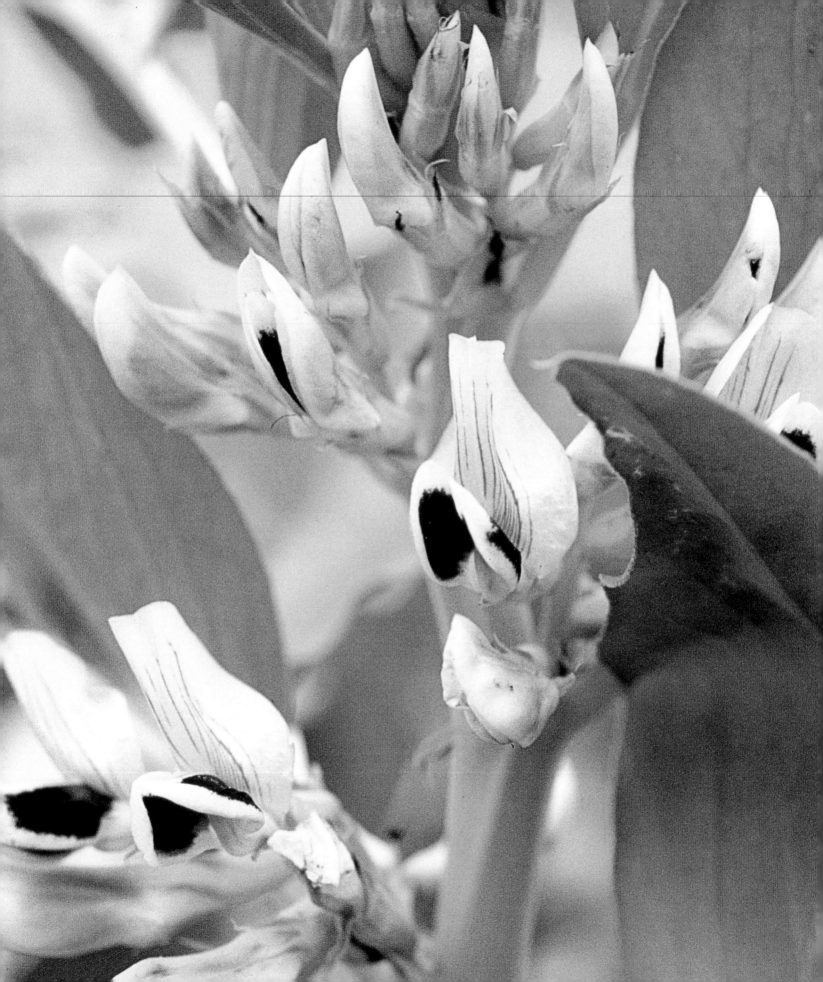

organic LIVING

Lynda Brown

A Dorling Kindersley Book

LONDON, NEW YORK, SYDNEY, DELHI,
PARIS, MUNICH, and JOHANNESBURG

Author's Dedication:
For Peter and Juliet

Senior Editor: Stephanie Farrow
Senior Art Editor: Jayne Jones
Art Editor: Vicki Groombridge
Project Editor: David Summers
DTP Designer: Conrad van Dyk
Production Manager: Maryann Webster

First American Edition, 2000
2 4 6 8 10 9 7 5 3 1

Published in the United States by
Dorling Kindersley Publishing, Inc.,
95 Madison Avenue, New York, NY 10016
First published in Great Britain in 2000 by
Dorling Kindersley Limited
9 Henrietta Street, London WC2E 8PS

A Pearson Company

DK Publishing offers special discounts for bulk
purchases for sales promotions or premiums.
Special editions, including personalized covers,
excerpts for existing guides, and corporate
imprints can be created in large quantities for
specific needs. For more information, contact
Special Markets Dept.,
Dorling Kindersley Publishing, Inc.,
95 Madison Ave., New York, NY 10016
Fax: (800) 600-9098.

A Cataloging-in-Publication record is available
from the Library of Congress

ISBN 0-7894-7193-0

Reproduced by Colourscan (Singapore)
Printed and bound in Italy
by Printer Trento S.r.l.

See our complete catalog at
www.dk.com

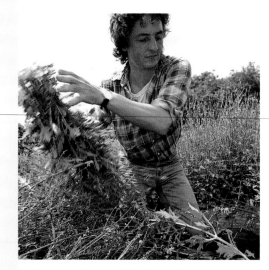

Introduction 6   The Complete
Organic Lifestyle 8

farming

food & drink

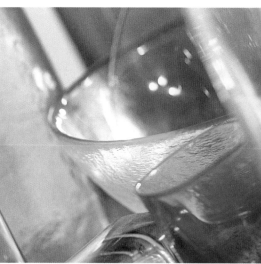

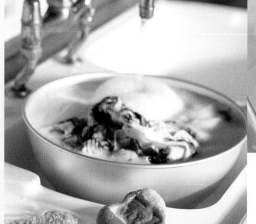

contents

baby care

health & beauty

gardening

home & office

organic directory

contributors

WINES & ALCOHOLIC BEVERAGES

Hilary Wright is an award-winning wine writer, widely
published in the field of organic wines. Previous books
include *Buying French Wine from the Chateau and
Vineyard*, *Buying Wine in France* and *Water into Wine*.

BABY CARE

Lizzie Vann MBE is the founder of the highly successful
organic children's food company, Organix. Her *Organic
Baby and Toddler Cookbook* is also available from
Dorling Kindersley.
Jill Barker has established the popular Green Baby
shop and mail order company in North London and is
an expert on the range of natural and organic products
available for babies.

HEALTH & BEAUTY

Josephine Fairley is a well-known beauty journalist with
a passion for organic health and beauty. She is Beauty
Editor of *The Mail On Sunday*'s *YOU Magazine*, and
writes for a wide range of women's magazines. Her books
include *The Beauty Bible* and *Feel Fabulous Forever*.

GARDENING

HDRA – the organic organisation is the UK's largest
organic membership organization. It promotes organic
gardening, farming, and food, researches improvements
in organic commercial growing and acts as a consultancy
for recycling and composting initiatives, organic garden
design, landscaping, and organic retailing and catering.

HOME & OFFICE

The Centre for Alternative Technology provides advice
and information on practical environmental solutions
through its visitor center in Wales and through a wide
range of publications, courses and an information service.
It also runs a consultancy service covering environmental
building, renewable energy and ecological sewage systems.

FABRICS & CLOTHING

Gina Moore runs Texture, an inspirational London shop
selling organic fabrics and goods, and has written for
books such as Dorling Kindersley's *Weekend Decorator*.

PETCARE

Christopher Day is a highly respected homeopathic vet
with a busy practice in Oxfordshire that uses organic and
eco-friendly animal care products. He has published
numerous books, including *The Holistic Management of
Dogs* and *The Homeopathic Treatment of Small Animals*.

Introduction

Welcome to the wonderful world of organics and a bright new start to your life.

Organic Living enables you to make positive, feel-good choices about every aspect of your life, from the food you eat to where you bank, and aims to help you to get more out of your life, easily and naturally, by making simple choices and changes for the better. Whether you choose to buy organic food, want the best start for your baby, go organic in your garden or choose more eco-friendly options in your home, we sincerely hope *Organic Living* will give you all the inspiration you need.

The organic way is about moving forward and finding new and better solutions. It is both visionary and pragmatic. At its heart, the message is very simple: respect nature,

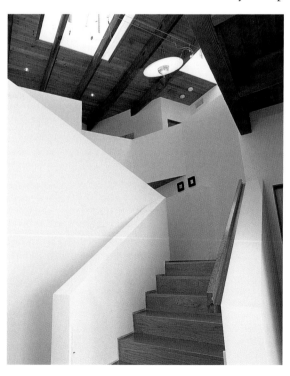

and nature will be your best friend; and cooperation at all levels, rather than destruction or domination, makes the best sense and bears lasting fruits. As millions of people worldwide are discovering daily, the organic way *is* the better way – better for us and for our environment – and offers a positive, modern, and progressive, sustainable blueprint for the world in which we live.

At the dawn of our new century we have everything to play and live for. Never before has consumer power been so important. As the debate over the genetic modification of our world has shown, we can shape the world we live in if we want to, and we can make our views and wishes count. What is so exciting is that we have so much choice, and that the organic option is now a

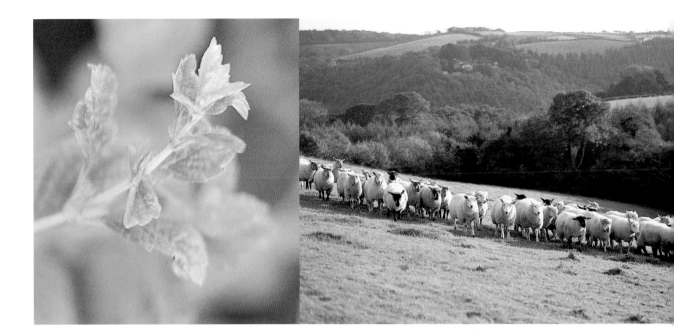

reality for everyone. Greener, cleaner, safer, and more socially responsible alternatives are now ours. The more we choose to buy into them and support the organic world, the happier and more secure our planet and everyone's future will be.

We are already well on our way. The world is going organic fast and the organic torch has been well and truly lit. Consumers are its torchbearers and are trailblazing the way. *Organic Living* celebrates this. We hope it brings you much enjoyment and a lifetime's organic health and happiness. Whoever and wherever we are, we and our planet deserve nothing less.

Happy organic living from all of us.

Lynda Brown

The complete organic lifestyle

In the sections that follow, we introduce you to what the organic lifestyle is all about, giving advice on where to start and on how you can make simple changes to your life for the better. Here you can read about some of the many inspiring producers, manufacturers, and entrepreneurs who are bringing organic life

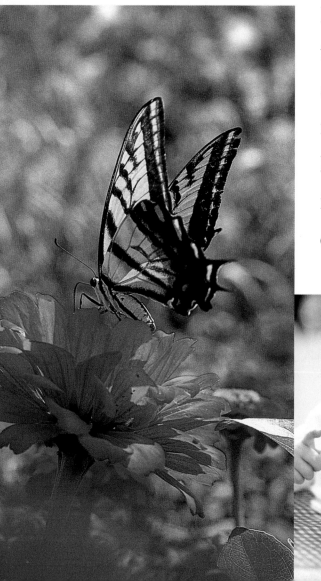

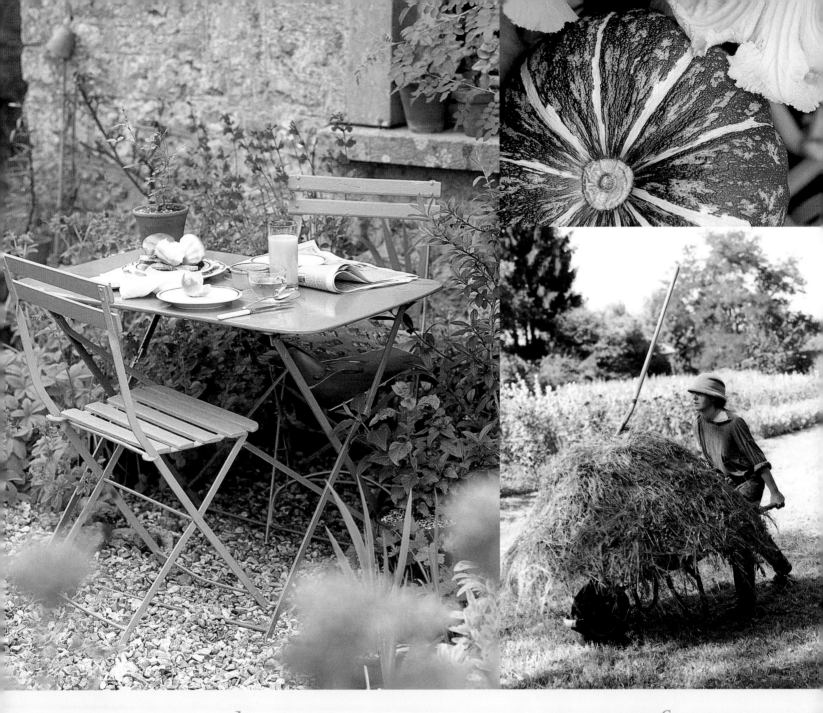

The more people who buy organic food, the more farmers will convert, and the more wildlife will benefit.

SIMON LYSTER, DIRECTOR GENERAL, THE WILDLIFE TRUSTS

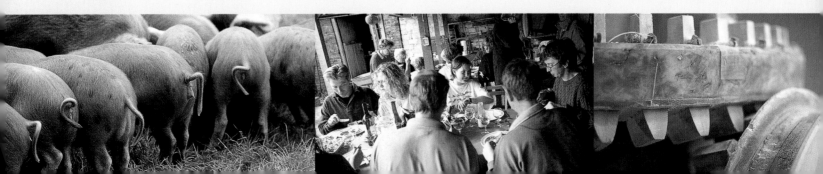

The complete organic lifestyle

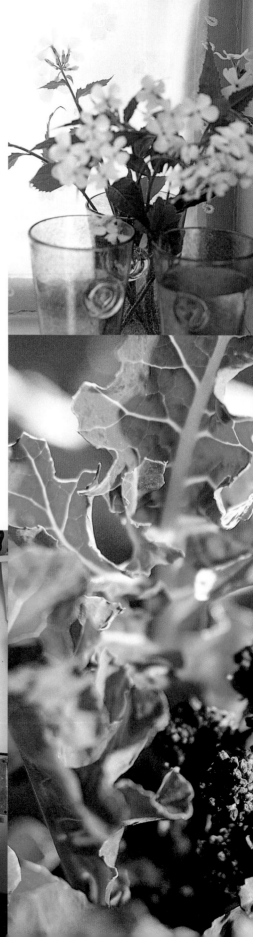

to our doorsteps. The organic lifestyle celebrates the naturally good things in life. You can eat, drink, wear, paint, and invest in organic. Organic living is a powerful force for change: we can be part of tomorrow's solutions rather than yesterday's problems. By buying into it, we each make a world of difference every time we

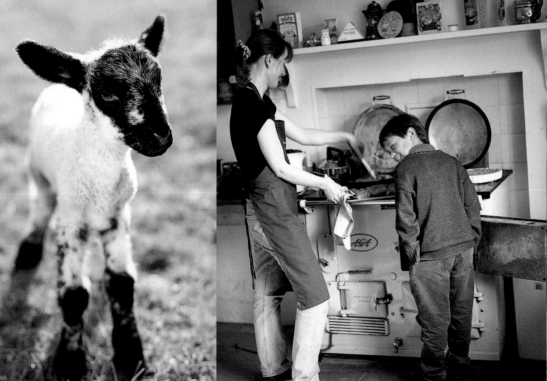

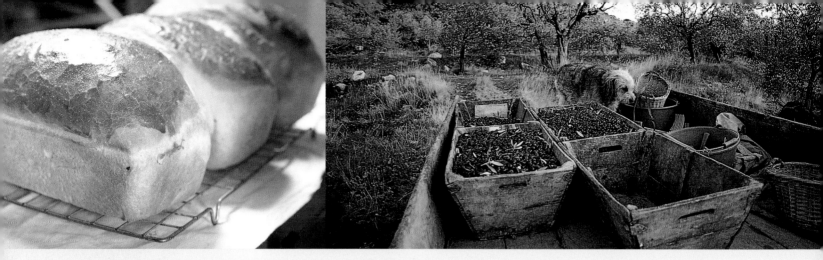

Following an organic lifestyle creates a better quality of life for you, those around you and the planet.

RENÉE J. ELLIOTT, FOUNDER, PLANET ORGANIC

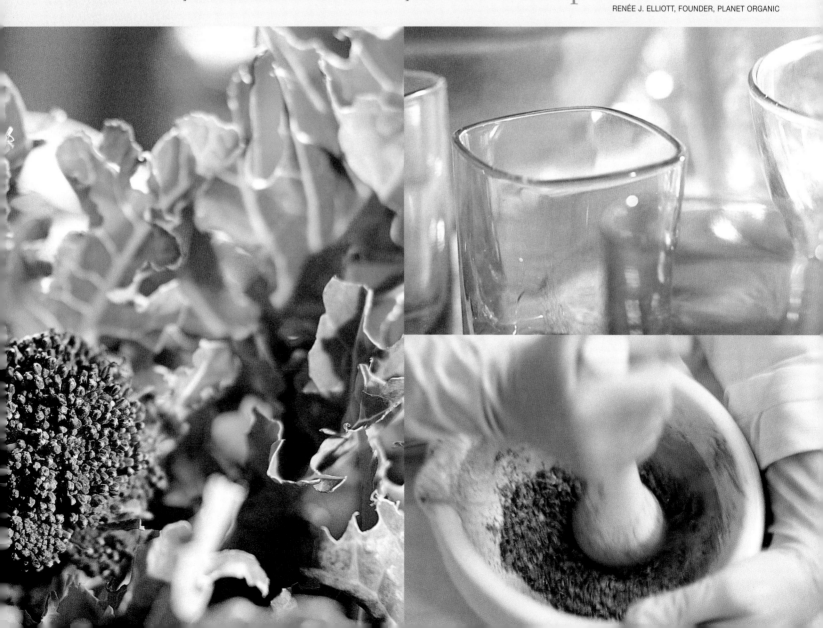

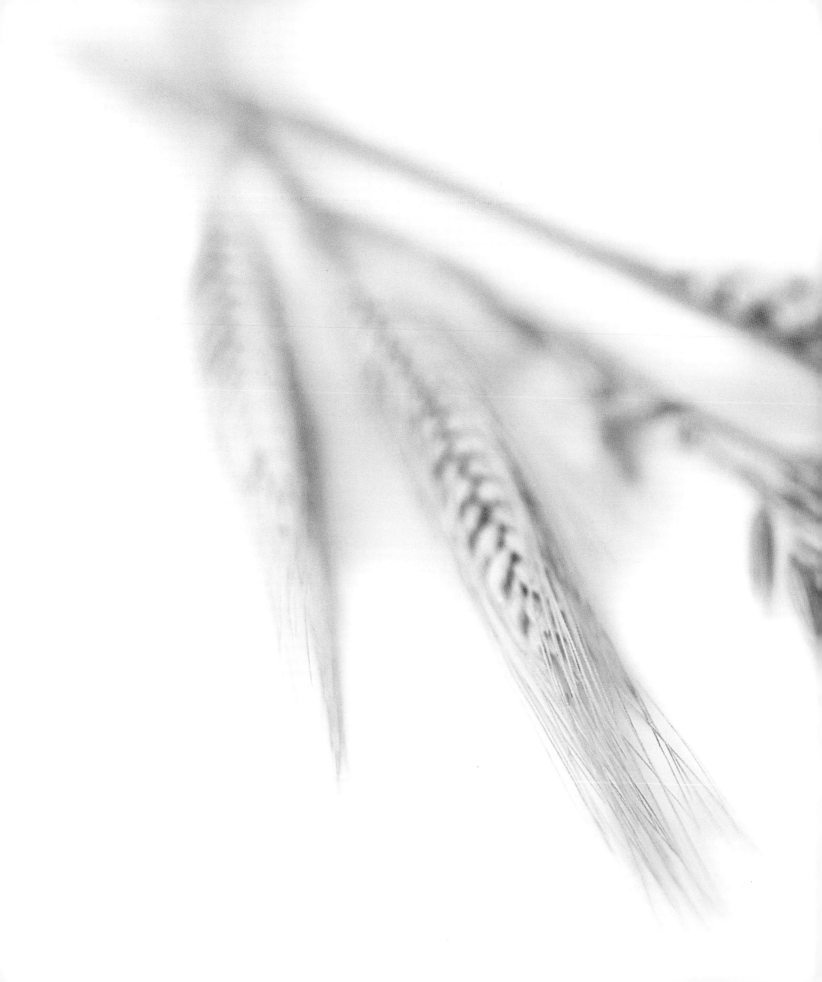

organic
FARMING

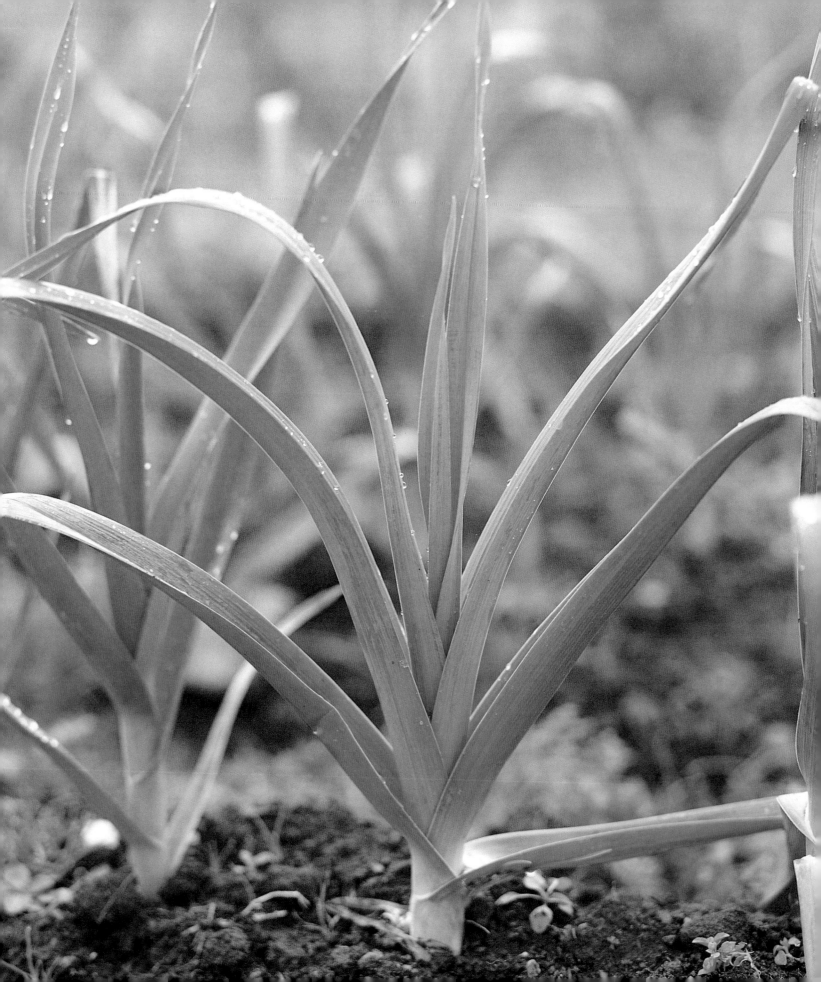

WHY GO organic

Going organic is better for you and better for the environment, since it is helping to reverse the ecological destruction that has been taking place since the middle of the 20th century.

By going organic and choosing eco-friendly options when you can, you will not only be helping to care for the environment in a wider sense and to limit the ecological damage that has taken place during recent years, but you will also become part of a social, economic, and environmental lifestyle that is finding fairer, more sustainable solutions for the future. Buying organic supports organic farming and the wide range of benefits it brings. Choosing the organic option also means supporting a system that campaigns against genetically modified (GM) crops and that is itself determined to be GM-free.

THE HEART OF THE MATTER

Organic farming is a system of agriculture that works in partnership with nature rather than against it. Unlike modern, industrialized agriculture, it does not seek to dominate or abuse natural systems, but to work in harmony with them. At its heart is the belief that agriculture is our primary healthcare system and that there is a direct link between the

health of the soil, that of the crops and animals raised on it, and ultimately that of the people fed and supported by it. This is why, for an organic farmer, it is health and vitality rather than yields that matter most. This means doing everything possible to nurture nature and to use farming practices that leave the environment in good shape.

A ROLE MODEL FOR THE FUTURE

Organic practices vary from country to country and organic farmers work in many different ways. All, however, share the same basic holistic aims and beliefs, based on respect for all living organisms. This approach embraces every aspect of cultivation and production, encouraging biodiversity and supporting local lifestyles. It also addresses wider eco-issues such as waste and energy conservation. In short, organic farming is the rock on which the foundations of the eco-lifestyle are built. Supporting it is the best way we can help to secure a better and healthier future for ourselves and the planet.

Organic farmers work with nature rather than against it

Nature is respected and protected

Biodiversity is encouraged

Animals are reared in humane conditions

Pollution is kept to a minimum

Secret of eternal life

As Franklin D. Roosevelt once said, the nation that destroys its soil destroys itself. The soil is the greatest environmental asset we have in the world, and healthy soil is fundamental to sustainable agriculture.

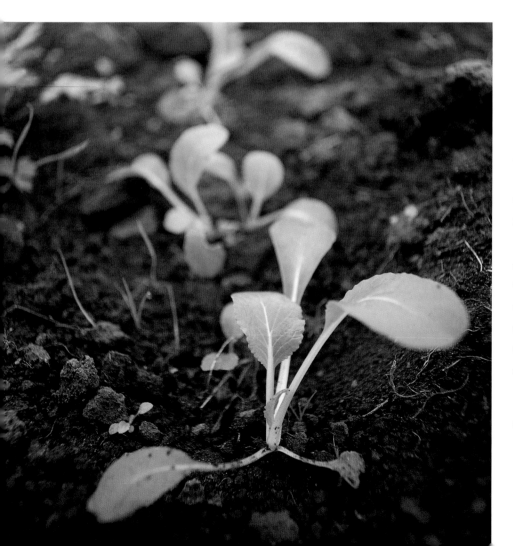

Take a brief look at this magical substance and it is easy to see why and how organic farming, which is based on maintaining rather than destroying soils, is so important for the future of the world. Organic farmers have long understood the value of healthy soil and know that good soil structure is crucial to the overall quality and health of their soil. Poor soil structure leads to increased soil erosion, which can cause ecological havoc with far-reaching consequences (*see far right*).

A WORLDWIDE WEB

Our soil comprises a soil-food web – a complex eco-system that involves animals, plants, insects, and microbes. In one gram of healthy soil, for example, there may be more than 10,000 species and a billion or more living organisms, most of

The fertility of the soil

which are microbes. It is these millions of soil bacteria and fungi, invisible to our eyes, that are especially important in breaking down nutrients, creating a living bridge between plant roots and minerals, and improving crop vigor and pest and disease resistance. Artificial fertilizers and pesticides have an adverse impact on the soil-food web, resulting in reduced nutrient cycling and crop vigor. Ironically, this leads to increased use of fertilizers and pesticides, forcing the whole soil eco-system into a spiral of decline.

WEIGHING UP THE EVIDENCE

The Rodale Institute in Pennsylvania has one of the longest-running Farming Systems Trials™ comparing organic and conventional agriculture in the world. Soils in the organic (*see below left*) and conventional (*see below right*) plots appear very different due to the higher level of soil organic matter present in the organically managed soils. Their research shows that organic soils not only have a better physical structure, with more biological activity and a larger, more stable balance of organic matter, but also retain water better and use nitrogen more efficiently than nonorganic soils.

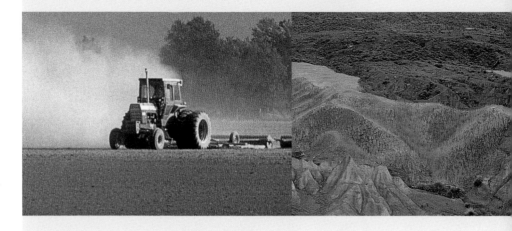

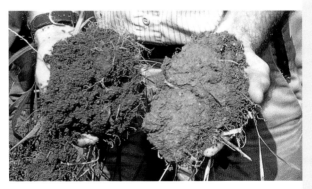

FEEDING THE WORLD: THE COST TO THE LAND

Since 1960 around 30 percent of the total crop land worldwide has been lost because of soil erosion by wind and water. In Mexico, for instance, it is estimated that only nine percent of the arable topsoil is left. Mechanized modern farming (*see above*) literally strip-mines the soil, weakening it forever, leaving it extremely vulnerable to permanent erosion by wind and water. One ecological consequence of this is that local agrochemical pollutants end up in rivers and oceans far away. The environmental group, Ecology Action, have calculated that, for every pound of food produced in this way in the US, up to 6 lb (2.75 kg) of soil are lost forever through wind and water erosion, while in China they estimate the loss is closer to 8 lb (18 kg) of soil per pound of food produced. In some areas, such as this devastated landscape in Bolivia (*see above right*), the land remaining has barely enough soil left to produce even a modest crop.

World's greatest disaster

"Soil erosion is one of the world's greatest disasters. It takes 500 years to form 1 in (2.5 cm) of topsoil, yet worldwide we are losing 75 billion tons of soil each year (13 tons of soil per person per year). The statistics are frightening. Mismanagement of soils due to poor agricultural practices costs the US alone $27 billion each year. If we want to grow food to feed the world, we need to radically rethink agriculture's abuse of natural resources and to start to care for our soils again. This is especially true when there are more than three billion malnourished people in the world today."

DAVID PIMENTEL, PROFESSOR OF ECOLOGY AND AGRICULTURAL SCIENCES, CORNELL UNIVERSITY, NEW YORK

is the future of civilization.

SIR ALBERT HOWARD, *THE SOIL AND HEALTH*, 1947

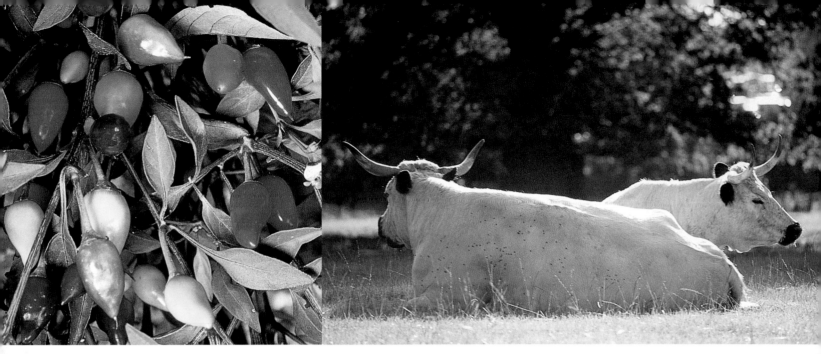

Embrace
biodiversity

Biodiversity literally means "living" diversity, and is derived from the ancient Greek word *bios*, or "life". It is our world's collective natural inheritance, belonging to no one in particular and to everyone in general.

Functioning as a natural bank of sustainability, biodiversity is the means by which our planet adapts, evolves, and regenerates itself. Until recently this rich reservoir was able to provide for all our basic necessities, such as food, water, shelter, and clothing, in addition to enriching our souls and imagination with its sheer wonder and variety. It is vital to preserve it for, without it, we are, quite literally, dead. Worldwide the wholesale destruction of biodiversity through intensive farming practices, industrial pollution, and abuse of pesticides, and the dramatic loss of many traditional crop varieties, is becoming critical. The threat of genetically modified crops and their impact on the planet's natural genetic pool is yet to be calculated. While modern, large-scale agriculture relies on standardization (with a consequent loss of biodiversity), the goal of

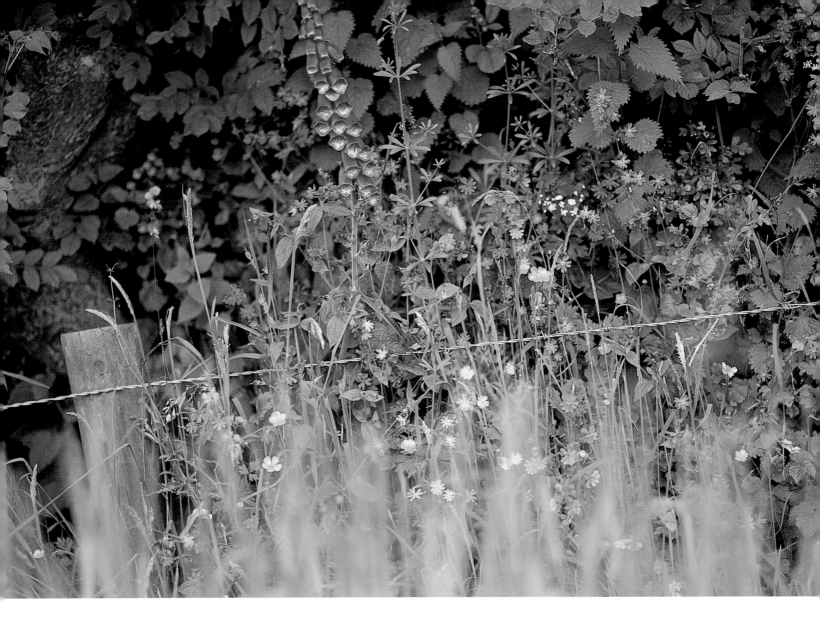

organic farms is to coexist with nature creating healthy and diverse eco-systems. The abundance of biodiversity is testament to their success.

VARIETY IS THE SPICE OF LIFE

On organic farms, measures to protect and improve biodiversity go hand in hand with conservation, and both are integral to organic standards. This means operating mixed farms with the widest diversity of crops or livestock possible, creating new habitats by planting indigenous trees and hedges, building beetle banks and ponds, and creating wild flower banks. Agricultural practices are adapted to ensure

maximum shelter for wildlife, so hedges are left to grow, wide field margins encourage wild flowers to flourish and create wildlife "corridors", and stubble is left on the fields to provide food and shelter for the birds. Organic farmers make use of traditional and local breeds of animals and crops, including beautiful species such as White Park cattle (*see top center*), the oldest breed in the UK, descended from the original wild white cattle that roamed the land 2,000 years ago. Unusual varieties of many fruits and vegetables, such as chilies (*see top left*), are also cultivated. This helps to ensure that genetic diversity is maintained.

EASY STEPS TO HELP PROTECT BIODIVERSITY

✤ Buy organic food (*see page 44*)

✤ Grow traditional and local varieties of plants in your garden (*see page 142*)

✤ Say NO to genetically engineered food and crops (*see page 30*)

✤ Join local and national wildlife and conservation organizations (*see page 223*)

Tools of the trade

Organic farming is a holistic system. Sustainable crop rotations, maintenance of biodiversity, and optimum crop health that is achieved by building soil fertility are the founding principles upon which it is based.

Rotations lie at the heart of soil fertility and good farm management

Soil fertility is built up with composted manures, homemade compost and green manures such as clover (*see right*)

Pests and diseases are kept in check using natural predators and preventative measures

Organic farming is as varied as nature itself and no two organic farms are ever the same. In conventional farming, artificial chemicals provide most of the answers; in organic farming, it is the farm itself and the way it is managed that counts.

Within conventional agriculture, dependency on regular inputs of artificial chemicals largely dictates how each farm is managed and also enables farming to become customized and highly specialized. On organic farms, the opposite is true. Organic farms are constantly changing and evolving, so organic farmers need to be creative and innovative, finding new solutions and techniques, and adapting to the seasons, the soil and the overall dynamics of their farms each year. The aim of organic farmers is to run their farm by working in harmony with nature rather than battling against it.

RINGING THE CHANGES

Rotating crops, animals and soil-enriching plants on the land, often in a five- or seven-year rotation cycle, lies at the heart of organic farming principles. Crops and animals are rotated to prevent disease buildup and soil imbalance. Green manures (*see page 154*) help build soil fertility. Clover leys (a short-term crop of grasses and clover) also provide first-class grazing for animals.

NATURAL ALLIANCES

Total control of pests and diseases is impossible, even with pesticides. On organic farms the aim is to keep pests and their natural predator populations in balance. Biodiversity and an absence of artificial pesticides help natural predators to flourish, so pests and diseases are

The health of man, beast, plant, and soil is one

usually far less of a problem on organic farms than on conventional ones. Farmers monitor their crops in the field more closely, time sowings to avoid major pest attacks, and choose resistant varieties. Organic farmers also have a different approach to weeds, using various control methods such as mulches or growing canopy crops. In some vineyards and orchards weeds provide protection for the soil and a habitat for natural predators. Annual weeds are never wasted, but are ploughed in or left on the ground to rot down naturally.

indivisible

Nurture nature

It has been proven without doubt that organic farming is good for the environment and wildlife. If you have a sound ecology, then everything thrives and is in balance.

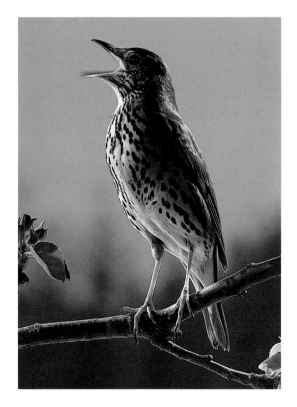

Organic farming offers the best blueprint for safeguarding our planet's biodiversity for future generations. Unlike conventional agriculture, protecting the environment, nurturing nature, practicing conservation techniques, minimizing pollution, and maximizing recyclable resources are not optional extras but an integral part of organic farming principles and standards. This is because, as organic farmers understand only too well, if you have a sound ecology, then the whole system thrives. Many of the techniques organic farmers use are very simple and are being taken up by "green" local authorities. They can be practiced in your own garden and home too (*see pages 144 and 176*).

LIVING CONSERVATION

Organic farms are havens for wildlife and for traditional species of wild flower such as corn cockle, poppies (*see above right*), corn marigold, and violets. Organic farmers treasure their ancient

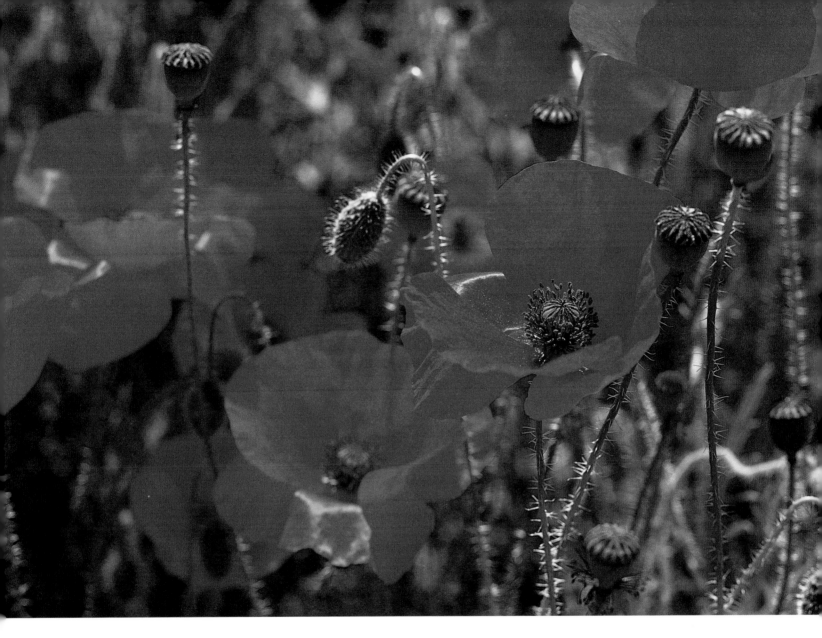

hedge banks, stone walls, meadows, woodlands, and other traditional habitats such as moorland, healthland and wetlands in the UK.

SAFE IN THEIR HANDS

Organic standards include conservation measures that protect these havens while improving the natural features of the land. Old farm buildings are protected and provide valuable wildlife habitats, especially for barn owls, bats, swallows, and house martins. Wide field margins provide shelter and food for the animals, birds, and insects they attract. Ponds are a valuable conservation resource and another magnet for wildlife, so organic farmers clear and maintain existing ponds and create new ones wherever possible. Ancient woodlands are prized as essential for preserving the landscape and diversity of the species. Planting native trees, taking the time to ensure that sowing, mowing, and harvesting cycles do not disturb ground-nesting birds and taking daily inspiration from nature's wonderful diversity are all part and parcel of an organic farmer's life.

Benign is best

"Intensive agriculture has had a catastrophic impact on wildlife over the last 50 years ... The only hope of reversing this trend is a radical change to more benign farming systems. The best farming system is organic."

SIMON LYSTER, DIRECTOR
GENERAL, THE WILDLIFE TRUSTS

Preventing pollution

Pollution of our land, water, and air, whether it is through toxic chemicals or intensive agricultural practices, is a modern scourge and a critical problem worldwide that affects everyone.

Every year there are an estimated 3 million acute pesticide-related poisonings, resulting in 220,000 deaths

Roughly 170 pesticides have been linked to major immune diseases such as cancer and allergies, and to infertility and problems in fetal development

Worldwide use of artificial nitrate fertilizer has grown by nearly sevenfold since the 1960s, yet it now ranks as a number one pollutant

In the US, insecticide use alone has increased tenfold, yet crop losses have almost doubled

Organic standards ban polluting practices and try to prevent pollution by not permitting the use of artificial fertilizers or pesticides. The standards also require that organic farmers do everything possible to minimize any unavoidable pollution and there are strict rules, for instance, governing the spreading of farmyard manures on the land and preventing any possible run-offs into water supplies.

MANURE MADNESS

Every year intensive livestock farming produces huge quantities of nitrogen-rich manure. Because artificial nitrogen is used to fertilize the land, and livestock is usually housed indoors, manure is regarded as a waste product and officially recognized as a serious disposal headache, since these "manure mountains" are often spread very heavily on small areas of land. This leaches high levels of nitrogen-rich discharges into the environment, polluting rivers and drinking water and posing a major threat to aquatic life. Organic farming frequently combines livestock and crops on the same farm. As a result, manure is a valuable resource. It is responsibly managed by composting and returned to the land in ways that cause minimal possible pollution.

NITROGEN NIGHTMARES

Artificial nitrates that superficially made the world a lush, green place and led to large increases in yields now rank as number one pollutants. Worldwide usage has increased by nearly sevenfold to 80 million tons per year, even though in developed countries crop yields reached a plateau in the 1980s and extra fertilizer applications have had no further effect. Around two thirds of the nitrogen fertilizers applied to crops do not get absorbed and leach into the environment, where they have devastating effects on local water systems and soil quality.

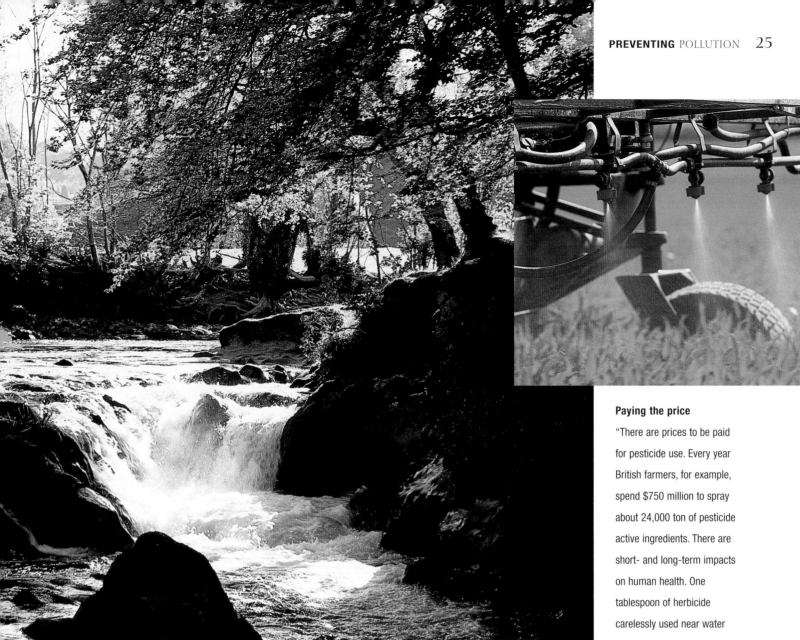

Paying the price

"There are prices to be paid for pesticide use. Every year British farmers, for example, spend $750 million to spray about 24,000 ton of pesticide active ingredients. There are short- and long-term impacts on human health. One tablespoon of herbicide carelessly used near water can pollute drinking water for 200,000 people. It costs $150 million every year to remove pesticides from water. Wouldn't it make more sense to pay farmers not to put pesticides into water rather than to pay water companies to remove pesticides from water?"

PETER BEAUMONT,
DEVELOPMENT DIRECTOR,
PESTICIDE ACTION NETWORK UK

PESTICIDE PERILS

Worldwide use and abuse of artificial pesticides, and the perils associated with it, makes for horrific reading. These highly toxic, hazardous, and invisible grim reapers of modern agriculture have invaded our land, seas, and air, and cause incalculable environmental damage, destroying biodiversity everywhere. Despite the fact that pest populations have risen, that pest and plants regularly develop resistance to pesticides, that pesticides once declared "safe" are repeatedly withdrawn or banned and that some persist in the eco-system for decades, each year we continue to pour another 5–6 billion lb (2–2.7 billion kg) of them into the environment. And we still lose as many crops now as before they were introduced. Pesticides are in our food, drinking water, and in the food chain at every level. The cocktail effect of ingesting tiny amounts of them has never been investigated: what we do know is the average daily diet now contains traces of thirty of them and that residues on individual food samples vary wildly.

Bursting with vitality

Organic farmers believe that growing crops organically provides the best possible way to produce healthy food. New research is now opening up the debate on crop health further.

Health as a birthright

"The birthright of all living things is health. This law is true for soil, plant, animal, and man; the health of these four is one connected chain."

SIR ALBERT HOWARD,
LIVING EARTH, 1954

Just as a person needs good nutrition and the right environment in order to flourish, so does a plant if it is to be healthy and radiate vitality. Though self-evident to many, until recently this and the potential consequences it may have for overall human health have been difficult to illustrate. New research in Switzerland, Denmark, and Germany by scientists developing a holistic approach to crop health is revealing some fascinating new insights that, if proven, may have far-reaching consequences.

THE APPLIANCE OF SCIENCE

We know that every plant is a living pharmacy full of thousands of chemical substances that are present in minute quantities, christened "secondary metabolites". Very little is known about these chemicals, but research in Denmark by Dr. Bodil Søgaard has found that one group of metabolites, the phenols, are antioxidants many times more powerful than vitamin C. Studies show that organic plants have a greater diversity and quantity of

phenols and, since nitrogen seems to suppress them, plants grown with artificial fertilizers have far fewer. One study at the Swiss Research Institute of Organic Agriculture (FiBL) showed that organic apple samples had over 18 percent more phenolic compounds than conventionally grown samples. Another study found much higher levels of phenols in organic wines than in their conventional equivalents. If these results are confirmed, the consequences for global agricultural systems that rely on nitrogen fertilizers could be significant.

GETTING THE PICTURE

Another exciting area of research uses advanced crystalization techniques. Studies involving analyses of hundreds of crystalization pictures (*see right*), show that those of organically and biodynamically grown food samples exhibit more regular patterns than their conventional equivalents. These studies have also shown that crystalization pictures of fresh organic foods have a more regular pattern

CRYSTAL CLEAR

Research being carried out in Switzerland by Dr. Ursula Balzer-Graf uses crystalization techniques to study conventionally, organically and biodynamically grown foods. Crystalization pictures (*see below*) are used to illustrate the "harmony of form" of plants, which is strongly affected by soil type, how the plants are fed and levels of nitrogen fertilization, as well as by variety, freshness and any processing involved. The example below compares an organically grown carrot with a conventionally grown carrot. The organic carrot sample is more regular and structured in form (*see top picture below*), while the conventional carrot sample is more fractured and fragmented (*see lower picture below*).

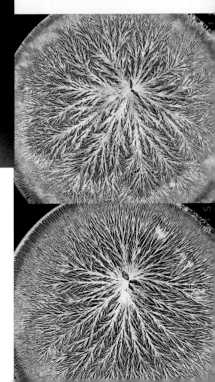

than processed organic foods, as do those of natural vitamin C compared with its synthetic equivalent. The implications of these differences and other related studies are not yet fully clear. What is clear, however, is that health cannot be measured in a test tube and that a holistic approach to crop health may deepen our understanding of the relationship between us, our soil, and our health and highlight the positive role that organic farming plays in ensuring that our food is as healthy as possible.

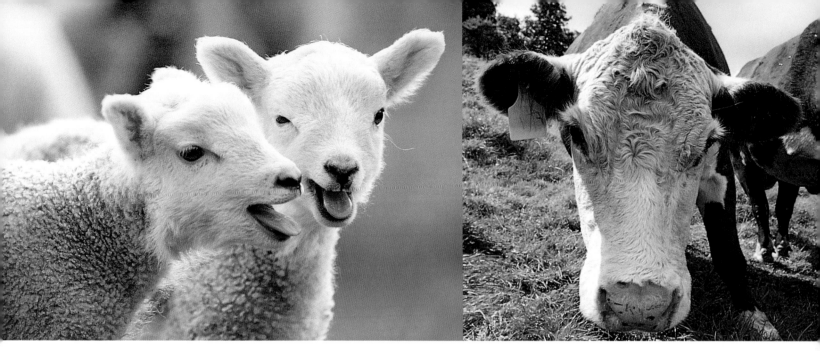

Be kind to animals

For an organic farmer, the natural health and welfare of his or her stock is paramount, and management practices are designed to keep animals as happy, healthy, and stress-free as possible.

Raising organic livestock is labor-intensive and requires considerable dedication and time, but ensures the livestock are as healthy and stress-free as possible. Organic farmers and their customers believe that this approach to animal welfare, in which the needs of the animal come first, is more satisfying for the farmer and the consumer, and results in better meat and dairy products. Animal welfare begins even before birth and, wherever possible, organic animals are raised on farms from closed herds (a closed herd is self-regenerating and retains its own female breeding stock). Any animals that are bought into a farm's herd must come from other organic farms (except day-old chicks) and have a full "audit trail" of traceability. Organic animals are reared on natural milk, not milk replacer, and are weaned at an older age than in conventional systems in order to build up their natural immunity.

ROOM FOR EXPRESSION

Intensive rearing methods and high stocking densities do not form part of the organic philosophy. Animals must have ample natural bedding and be given conditions that allow them to express their natural behavior. Generally, organic animals spend much of their time outside and many farmers keep their animals in family groups.

NATURALLY NURTURED

Organic animals graze exclusively on organic pastures and are fed only appropriate, natural, non-GM feeds, all or most of which must be organic. Animals on organic farms receive no routine antibiotics, wormers, or other medication, and all synthetic growth-promoting agents are prohibited (*see right*). Good health is maintained through good feeding and husbandry, and natural and homeopathic remedies are encouraged.

HAPPIER ENDINGS

Wherever possible, animals from organic farms are slaughtered in locally. The maximum time allowed for traveling to a slaughterhouse is eight hours. Provision for food and water must be given, and animals are slaughtered in small numbers. To avoid contamination or accidental mixup with other, non-organic carcasses, organic animals are usually the first to be killed and they must be identifiable at all times. With the exception of poultry (as one-day-old chicks), only animals that have been born and raised on organic holdings are allowed to be sold as organic meat, and must have a comprehensive audit trail of traceability from farm to table.

The need for compassion

"Sadly, as the European Union begins to abandon some of the most cruel factory farming systems, we find them entrenched in North America and growing rapidly and unsustainably in Asia. Already China has turned from being a grain exporter to being a grain importer – not to feed its people, but to feed the pigs in its burgeoning factory farms. The world simply cannot sustain feeding such a huge and growing proportion of its cereals and oilseeds to intensively farmed animals."

JOYCE D'SILVA,
DIRECTOR, COMPASSION
IN WORLD FARMING

ROUTINE ANTIBIOTICS – THE CASE AGAINST

Rearing animals intensively puts unnatural stresses on them. As a result they are more likely to become ill, and so are frequently or routinely dosed with antibiotics to prevent and treat disease. In addition, antibiotics are also used extensively as growth promoters, so that most intensively reared cattle and virtually all growing pigs and broiler chickens (*see below*) receive them in their feed throughout their lives. Growth-promoting antibiotics also kill most natural bacteria in farm animals but not all strains of salmonella. The incidence of food poisoning from salmonella is still rising, and the strains of bacteria responsible for this are routinely found in intensively farmed animals. Overuse of antibiotics in this way is resulting in widespread bacterial resistance to antibiotics, causing the development of new strains of disease that are not treatable with current antibiotics and pose a continuing threat to human health. Routine use of these valuable medicines is banned in organic farming, and the UK's Soil Association is leading the campaign to stop this practice in future (source: The Soil Association, *The Use and Misuse of Antibiotics in UK Agriculture*, 1999).

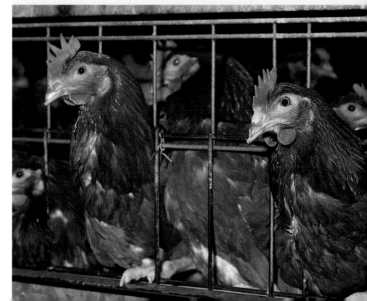

The voice of reason

Genetic engineering is the single most important issue of our lifetime. It raises questions on many different levels, including environmental, social, ethical, and political.

The choice

"Industrial, intensive farming now faces a choice between escalating its war on nature by embracing GM technology, or changing direction, to work with the grain of nature. Corporations are desperate for the profits GM products will bring them, but we decide what we want to buy. Scientists find rearranging nature very exciting, but we have to decide between right and wrong. And in a historic victory over big science and big business, people worldwide are saying no to GM food. This is a victory for civilized values and for all who enjoy good, healthy food."

PETER MELCHETT, EXECUTIVE DIRECTOR, GREENPEACE

For many scientists, genetic engineering offers the ultimate prize: control of life itself and an Aladdin's cave of scientific possibilities. For the agrochemical and pharmaceutical companies, it offers undreamed-of profits and domination of the world's food and seed supply. For intensive farmers, it offers a new technological quick-fix to the problems that nitrates and pesticides were supposed to solve but have not.

It is also the biggest gamble we have ever taken, which – if it goes wrong – could have devastating consequences for our health and our planet. Once released, genetically modified organisms (GMOs) can never be recalled – that is the problem. At the heart of these issues lies a debate on democracy and fundamental human rights, on who "owns" nature, and on whether, as the UK's Prince of Wales argues, by tampering with nature in this way we are entering realms that belong to God alone.

BEYOND THE POINT OF RETURN

The genetic engineering genie is already out of the bottle. The question is: what do we use it for, and who should own and control it? Its use in medicines – to find treatments for previously incurable conditions, for example – for consenting individuals in properly controlled and closed conditions is a very different matter from the colonization of the environment with "Frankenstein" crops that could never exist outside a laboratory and whose long-term effects are unknown. There is no doubt, too, that although consumers have said a resounding NO to GM foods, we and our children continue to be used as unwitting guinea pigs, and our environment continues to be used as an open-air laboratory. Many animal feeds already contain GM corn (*see page 56*) or soy (*see page 100*), many cosmetics and health supplements have been produced using GM

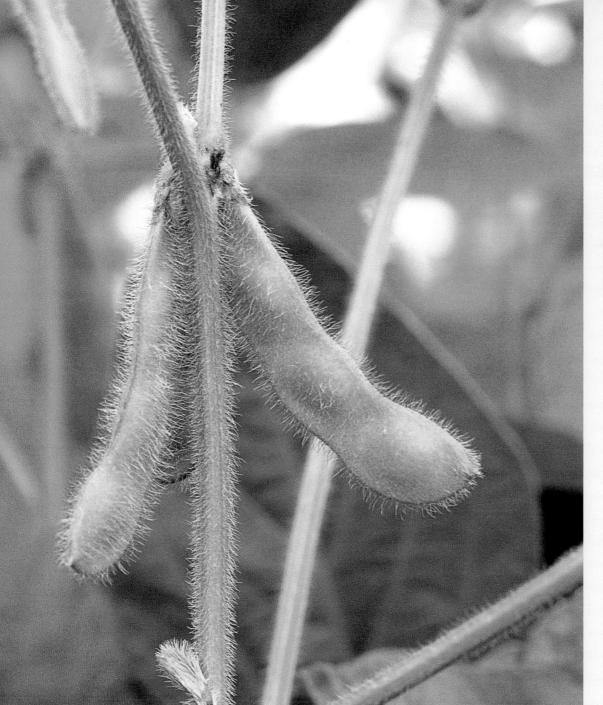

THE HIDDEN DANGERS
GM derivatives are already present in many products (*see below*), and GM crop trials are already polluting the environment.

WHAT IS BEING GENETICALLY ENGINEERED
Not only...

❖ Animals

❖ Bacteria

❖ Coffee

❖ Cosmetics

❖ Cotton

❖ Drugs

❖ Fish

❖ Food crops such as corn and soy (*see left*)

❖ Livestock feeds

❖ Trees, lawns, plants, and seeds

❖ Vines

❖ Vitamins

But also...

❖ Biological weapons

❖ Contraceptives

❖ Humans (germ-line therapy on embryos, which is still in its infancy)

❖ Plastics, starches, and industrial chemicals

derivatives. GM field crop trials are already polluting the environment; many beekeepers, for example, can no longer guarantee that their honey is GM-free (*see page 96*). The question we have to ask is: is this right? The organic movement has said that GM crops have no place in organic agriculture and it offers people the *only* realistic non-GM choice. Is it right that all farmers who wish to stay GM-free are threatened too? The outcome of this debate will determine the world we shall inhabit – and inherit – for ever more. Choosing the organic option, and supporting organizations that campaign for the right to say NO, will help to ensure that the world gets the breathing space it deserves.

MAPPING OUT ORGANICS

The organic revolution is happening worldwide and providing a powerful force for agricultural change everywhere. Demand for organic food is at an all-time high: global growth is expected to reach up to 20 percent each year for the next decade or more, and to account for between two and five percent of all food sales worldwide.

north america

United States of America

The number one organic producer worldwide, with 1.4 million acres (5,670 sq km) of certified organic farmland. The annual rate of market growth is 15–20 percent, with the market currently worth $6.6 billion and expected to rise to more than $13 billion by 2003. Major exports: fruit and vegetables, grain, and animal feeds and processed products.

central & south america

Cuba

Organic agriculture was adopted as part of its official policy in 1990. Growing for domestic consumption, Cuba had become self-sufficient in basic vegetables and fruit by 1996 and more than 80 percent of its pest control had become based on biological controls.

Mexico

High-quality Mexican organic coffee is a favorite with European coffee drinkers. Major exports: coffee, fruit, avocados, and vegetables.

Brazil

Organic production is steadily increasing. Brazil is a major source of non-GM soy. In 1999 the state of Rio Grande do Sol made history by banning all field trials of GM soy and prohibiting any GMO releases in the state. Other states in Brazil are attempting to follow suit. Major exports: fruit and soy.

Argentina

A rising star: 85 percent of Argentinean organic crops are exported, including organic beef. Several major new fruit plantations have been set up and further expansion is planned. Exports: flax, sunflower seeds, apples and pears, citrus fruits, olive oil, and wine.

europe

Denmark

Nearly 50 percent of households buy organic foods and organic milk is the norm. Major exports: pork and dairy products.

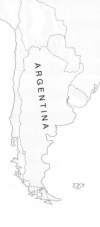

africa

Egypt

Organic agriculture began here in 1978, when a biodynamic farm was established in the desert. Since then more than 180 organic farms have been set up. Major exports: vegetables, including early new potatoes, cotton, and medicinal herbs.

Burkina

Each year 10,000 mango growers in Burkina produce 50,000 tons of organic mangos for export to Europe fresh or as dried mango slices. Its other major export crop is organic sesame seeds.

Tanzania

Many organic farming initiatives are being developed. Tanzanian honey is one of the oldest fairly traded products available. Major export: honey.

POLAND

HUNGARY

EGYPT

TANZANIA

MADAGASCAR

C H I N A

INDIA

JAPAN

asia

India

All types of organic food produced for the domestic market. Much of India's biodiversity has already been destroyed. In the 1950s more than 30,000 varieties of rice were grown in India. Today seed-saving initiatives such as the Navdanya Project attempt to secure the remaining 600 varieties. Main exports are tea, coffee, spices, nuts, cotton, and herbal cosmetics.

China

A large area of central China has just been earmarked for organic production. Currently has 10,000 acres of certified organic land producing more than 30 types of organic produce for export. Due to consumer demand, China's first organic shops are opening in Shanghai.

australasia

Australia

The land area under organic cultivation is currently 4.2 million acres, and is set to double within 10 years. The country's biggest export market is Japan, especially for organic beef. Production of organic wine is steadily increasing. Vegetables are a major organic crop, as are oil and grain crops.

A U S T R A L I A

New Zealand

Organic food and farming is the fastest-growing sector of the market, and the area of land farmed organically is expected to increase to 30 percent by 2010. Major exports: kiwi fruits, apples, and processed vegetables. New Zealand also produces organic avocados, wine, and citrus fruits.

NEW ZEALAND

Madagascar

An organic paradise, producing organic coffee, cocoa, pineapples, honey, vegetables, vanilla, herbs, coconuts, and palm oil, all for the export market.

Japan

The organic market is currently worth $2.5 billion dollars and is growing fast. About 2.5 percent of agricultural land is already under organic cultivation. Demand out-strips supply. Imports are largely from New Zealand, Australia, and the US. Roughly 40 percent of the population belong to a natural food buyers' cooperative.

Cook Islands

Plans to be the first nation in the world to go totally organic by 2003.

Sweden

Over 10 percent of agricultural land is already organic, and the country is on target for 20 percent by 2005. Major exports: meat (especially pork) and dairy foods.

Germany

The largest organic market in Europe, accounting for one third of all European organic meat and dairy products, and second only to the US worldwide, with over 8,000 organic producers, the highest per capita consumption of organic food and drink in Europe, and, after Italy,

the second largest land area in Europe under organic cultivation and in conversion. Exports: beer, meat, dairy foods, processed foods, baby foods, condiments, and cosmetics.

Switzerland

With over 7 percent of land area (4,500 farms) already under organic cultivation, organic farming and food are major growth markets. Main production is dairy products; 25 percent of the milk sold by a

major Swiss supermarket chain is organic, which expects that 20 percent of all its product categories will be organic in the near future.

United Kingdom

The UK has the fastest-growing organic market in Europe. An Organic Food and Farming Targets Bill proposes a target of 30 percent agricultural land and 20 percent of food consumed to be organic by 2010. Currently just over 1 percent of land is farmed organically. Demand far outstrips supply and 70 percent of organic products are imported.

Hungary

In Hungary exports of organic food have doubled to over $12 million, and organic agriculture is helping to revitalize rural areas. Exports: grain, herbs, and vegetables.

Poland

Organic agriculture is playing a major role in rebuilding the rural economy. Much of the soft fruit

used for flavoring yogurts, jam, and other processed fruit products sold in Europe comes from Poland. Exports: wheat and soft fruits.

Italy

Exponential growth in organic production means Italy has more than 15,000 organic farms. The temperate Mediterranean climate makes it ideal for a wide range of crops. Major exports: pasta and pasta products, peaches, apricots, grapes, zucchinis, tomatoes, olive oil, and wine.

Spain

One of Europe's largest producers and exporters of organic food, which exports over 90 percent of its organic production. It has more than 865,000 acres of organic land and around 12,000 organic producers. Olive oil is the leading organic product, accounting for more than 40 percent of organic land. Major exports: olive oil, fruit, and vegetables.

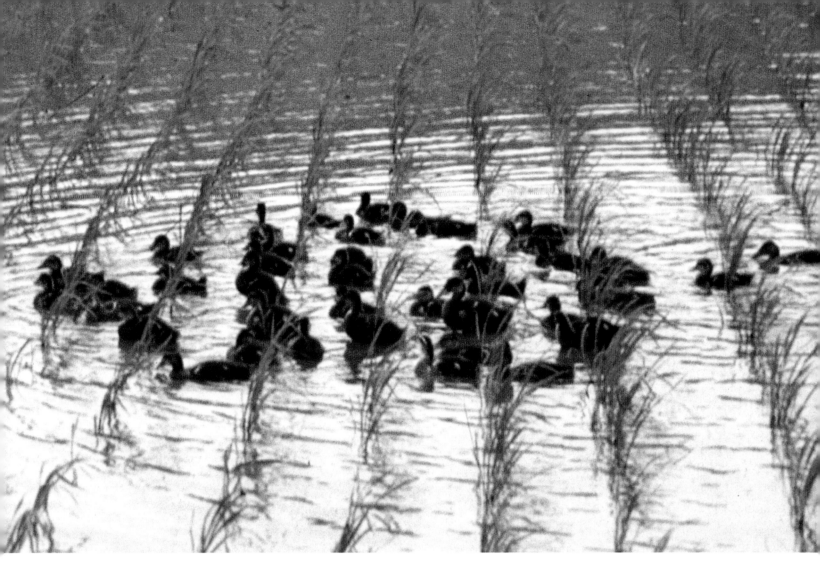

Organics
around the world

Large and small organic farmers, individuals and cooperatives, pioneers, and traditionalists – all share the same vision of growing healthy food and making eco-friendly products in ways that will sustain us and our planet.

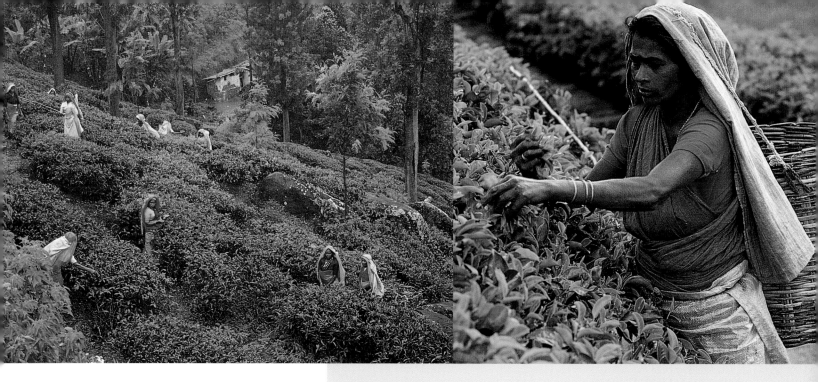

Ripe, fresh dates from California, sugar cane grown under the blue skies of Mauritius, fragrant teas from Sri Lankan hillsides, fruity olive oils from traditional Spanish olive groves, rare coffees from Papua New Guinea, heady organic wines from New Zealand – organic food and drink comes from all corners of the globe and stands for quality and enjoyment. Pure, natural lotions, potions, and soaps can help to keep you clean. Soft organic cotton clothing and bedding, and beautiful furniture and floors made with wood from sustainable forests, can add another dimension to your home. The richness of diversity, as shown below, is a crucial defining element that sets organic farmers apart from the rest. Knowing that what you buy comes from real individuals, whose daily efforts enrich the world in which we live, is a treasure we can all rejoice in, and something to be celebrated every time we shop.

THE DUCK PATROL

Introducing ducklings into rice paddy fields (*see above left*), the brainchild of Mr. Furuno, a small organic farmer in Fukuoka, Japan, has revolutionized the lives of thousands of peasant

TIME FOR TEA

The Iddalgashinne biodynamic tea estate (*see above*) is set in breathtaking scenery, 6,500 ft (2,000 m) above sea level in the Beragala Hills of the Uva district in Sri Lanka. Protected by virgin rainforests, this is a beautiful green jumble of biodiversity that produces top notch teas. The estate has a workforce of 1,400 people, its own nursery school, house-building programs and three medical centers. It is currently in transition to community ownership under the "Social Action Plan" program.

As a biodynamic plantation, the growers use a lunar calendar to help them determine the best time for operations such as planting and pruning. They also use specific biodynamic preparations made on the estate to treat the tea bushes and soil. Worms are supplied with green manures and coconut waste to generate compost for the tea bushes. Other worms are fed with beneficial herbs to produce "worm bath water" that is applied in tiny, homeopathic quantities as a plant tonic. The tea is hand-picked and hand-rolled according to traditional practices in the plantation's own tea factory.

Sri Lanka produces other organic teas of remarkable quality. The island as a whole does not use pesticides, except as a spot treatment, and has been leading the way in natural predator control since the 1960s by encouraging beneficial insect populations with measures such as growing sunflowers and providing shaded areas for wasps that attack the Tortrix moth.

Organics around the world

Rights & wrongs

"There is a misconception that organic farming is the same as subsistence or 'traditional' farming. Nothing is further from the truth. Organic farming is modern, progressive, and a blueprint for sustainability. It is the wrong strategy to try and feed the world by depleting the soil, polluting the environment, or introducing genetic engineering. We must ensure that people can feed themselves ... only organic farming has the right approach to this and seeks to find solutions that last."

BERNWALD GEIER, DIRECTOR, INTERNATIONAL FEDERATION OF ORGANIC AGRICULTURAL MOVEMENTS

farmers in southeast Asia. The ducklings do the weeding, and they eat insects and other pests . They also oxygenate the water as they paddle, helping to make the rice plants grow strong, as does the natural fertilizer of the ducklings' droppings. Once the rice is ready to harvest, the ducks are removed and fattened up on waste rice grains from the rice-polishing plant. After laying eggs, which are hatched to provide more ducklings for the next season, the ducks are sold, providing extra income for the farmers. Except for the small amount of waste rice grain, they are entirely self-sustaining. Yields have increased by 20–50 percent using this method, weeding time saved is 240 person-hours per acre, and farmers' incomes have doubled. Each year Mr. Furuno's farm of about two acres produces about seven tons of rice, 30 ducks, 4,000 ducklings, and enough vegetables to support 100 people. He has not patented his method and shares his ideas freely through videos, lectures, and teaching.

CRIMSON TIDE

American growers are restoring their cranberry bogs to their former glory – organically. Cranberries are native to North America and used to grow wild until cultivated varieties were developed, spawning a multi-million dollar business. At Cranberry Hill Organic Farm, in Massachusetts (*see below left*), the farmers grow traditional cranberry varieties and preserve their natural habitat, which provides a refuge for birds, insects, and pond life. It is hard work all year round. During the coldest winter month the bogs are flooded with clean spring water to protect the cranberry vines from cold. Sand is then spread to help the vines root more easily. In late spring, the bogs are flooded again for 30 days to retard pests and weeds, and throughout the summer the bogs are hand-weeded. Unlike conventional cranberry producers, organic growers use no pesticides and feed vines only with organic nutrients. In the autumn the berries are harvested with wooden scoops and picking machines, then cleaned, sorted, and packed on site. They are sold fresh throughout the US and are beginning to appear in Europe as well as in Japan and Taiwan. Organic cranberries are also dried and juiced for use all year round.

THE PIG TALE

At the Herrmannsdorfer Landwerkstätten, near Munich in Germany, the link between farmer and consumer is

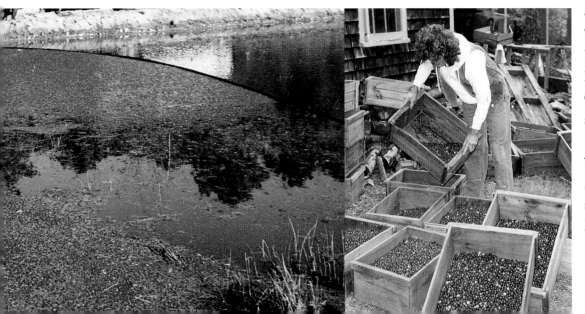

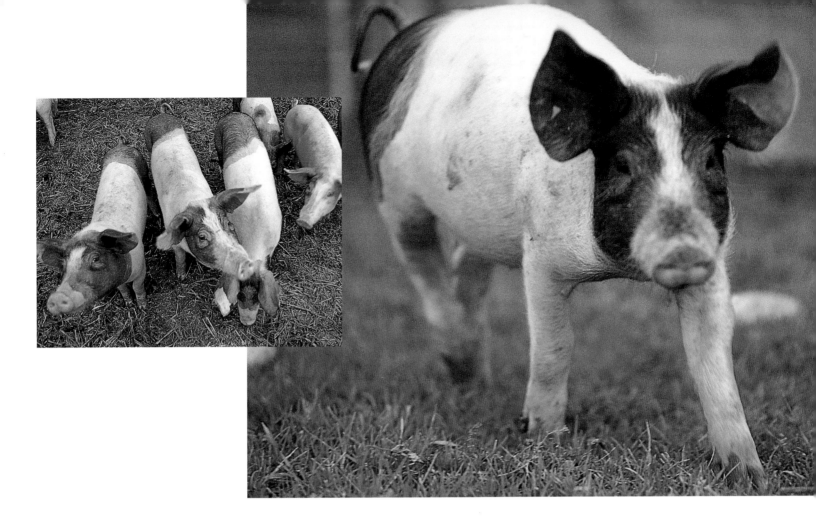

This is about us, about our health, our vitality, our environment, and our children's environment.

KARL LUDWIG SCHWEISFURTH, FARMER, HERMANNSDORFER LANDWERKSTÄTTEN

complete. The pigs roam outside in good weather, retiring to stalls when the conditions are bad. About 15–30 pigs share a stall, grouped according to age. They lead a happy life and are treated with respect and care. The pigs feed on leftovers from other operations on the farm, such as unsold bread from the shop, scraps from the restaurant, and mash from the beer-making process. Animals are slaughtered humanely on site and processed immediately to make the farm's acclaimed, preservative-free sausages, liverwurst, salamis, and traditionally cured hams, which are served in their own restaurant or sold in their farm shop and in other local shops and supermarkets. The owner of this inspirational farm, the pioneering Karl Ludwig Schweisfurth, aims to run a "zero emission" farm where everything is recycled. All organic waste, including that from the pigs, goes to a Biogas recycling plant, where bacteria purify its liquid content back into clean water and transform the nonliquid waste into fertilizer, which is plowed back into the land, and methane gas, which powers a generator to produce heat and electricity.

Looking local going

Foods and goods produced locally offer a sustainable way forward. Buying organic and fair-trade foods and goods (*see page 220*) helps local communities to flourish and is something in which all of us can become involved.

LOCAL FOOD LINKS

There are many ways you can get involved in the Go Local programs (*see also page 234*).

❖ Boxed food plans

❖ Farmers' markets

❖ Farm shops

❖ Women's Institute markets

❖ Food cooperatives

❖ City farms, community gardens, and orchards

❖ Subscription farms and community-owned farms

❖ Local food directories

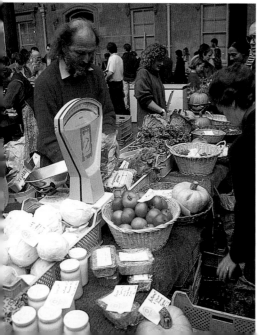

Food produced and consumed locally can be fresher, healthier, and more economical than produce that has been transported for long distances, and often has less packaging too. Buying local produce helps communities to thrive, restores trust, and re-connects consumer to farmer. It lets buying food be a pleasurable and meaningful experience again.

The Go Local movement is a worldwide initiative that involves national and local campaigns as well as community and farming projects. Find out about local food links and boxed food plans (*see left*). Contact your tourist board or local authority and ask for their local food directory.

Supermarkets are also starting to stock local food – ask yours to do the same.

GLOBAL GO LOCAL

Local and sustainable food links are developing in many countries. Farmers' markets (*see left*), for example, began in the US in the 1970s and have been a roaring success. There are now more than 2,500 of them here in the US, generating over $1 billion annually for growers. The Seikatsu Club, an organic consumer cooperative in Japan set up by a group of Japanese women, now has 153,000 members. The Bio Co-op consumer cooperatives in France, started in 1987, are run by and for local organic consumers, with more than 160 branches.

"PLANT A SEED AND GROW A COMMUNITY"

In the past farms have usually been under private ownership. Now projects such as subscription farming and community farms in cities and in rural areas enable people to get actively involved, to become social investors and to reap a share of the harvest. Already well established in the US and Japan, subscription farming is a variation on boxed food plans where you pay in advance for a share of the harvest, which is then divided up as a weekly box. Members also help with growing, harvesting, and packing. Community-owned farms are variation popular in many countries. These allow you to part-own a local farm by buying a modest amount of shares. Members can help with the day-to-day running of the farm, which is owned cooperatively. City farms and community gardens are run for and by local communities and bring the country to the city. They range from

global

nature gardens, ecological parks, and allotments (*see below*) to demonstration city farms. All provide a haven for wildlife and a green focus for local communities, especially children. Many grow and sell their own organic produce. The UK, for example, has over 250, involving over 300,000 local people and attracting 3 million visitors a year.

By supporting organic farmers, we will be able to create a sustainable future for ourselves and our planet.

HELEN BROWNING OBE, CHAIRMAN, THE SOIL ASSOCIATION

The natural food link

Organic farms all over the world provide living proof that organic farming works. Duchy Home Farm, on the Prince of Wales's Highgrove Estate in the UK, is one of the many thousands that provide daily inspiration for us all.

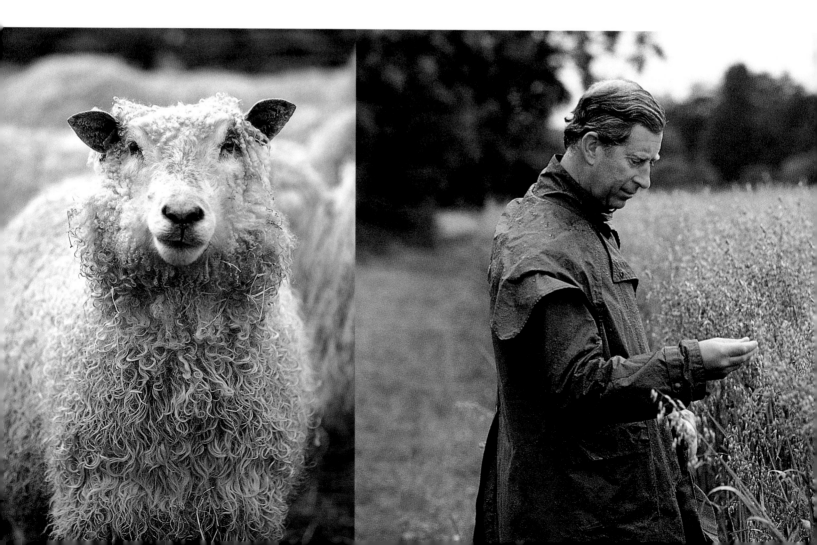

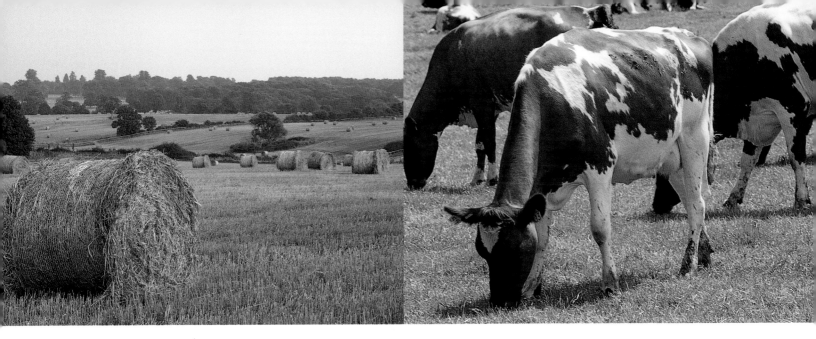

The Prince of Wales is one of Britain's best-known organic farmers. Like many thousands of people who care about the environment and believe we have a responsibility to look after our planet, he has spoken out and championed environmental causes for over thirty years. He began converting the Duchy Home Farm (*see above and left*) at Highgrove, Gloucestershire, in 1986, and today it is fully organic, providing high-quality food for the local community and beyond.

THE PRINCE'S ORGANIC EXAMPLE

Like every organic farm, Duchy Home Farm works with, rather than against, nature. Permanent grass strips 6½ ft (2 m) wide that surround every field, and acres of new broadleaf woodland, along with hedges that create new green lanes, ensure an abundance of natural predators. To further protect biodiversity, the farm keeps six rare breeds: Hebridean and Cotswold sheep (*see far left*), Large Black pigs, and Gloucester, Irish Moiled and Aubrac cattle.

As an organic demonstration farm, Duchy Home Farm is visited regularly by farmers wanting to convert to organic methods, as well as by scientists and politicians. Independent research

has confirmed that – like countless other organic farms – the Prince's organic farm is more beneficial to wildlife, causes less pollution and, once conversion is complete, is more profitable than similar conventional farms.

DEVELOPING THE NATURAL FOOD LINK

Duchy Home Farm's organic produce is distributed widely. Its organic vegetable box program supplies 150 local families each week. Milk from the farm, which is sold through the Organic Milk Suppliers Co-operative (OMSCo; *see page 77*), finds its way into Yeo Valley yogurts and Alvis Brothers cheese. Duchy Home Farm's rye is taken to nearby Shipton Mill for milling and from there on to be made into organic bread. Its lamb and beef are sold through local and national butchers and the Organic Meat Co-operative, and its pork is used to produce Duchy Originals organic bacon and sausages. This organic and natural food and beverage brand, launched by the Prince in 1992, was set up to facilitate the production of the highest-quality food and drink products. All its profits are donated to the Prince's Charitable Foundation. The range also features Duchy Originals award-winning organic cookies.

Health & naturalness

"The objectives for the agriculture of the 21st century must surely embrace a wide definition of sustainability… which stresses the virtues of health and naturalness throughout the food chain; and which will enhance the quality of life."

HRH THE PRINCE OF WALES 1996, IN HIS LADY EVE BALFOUR LECTURE (COMMEMORATING THE 50TH ANNIVERSARY OF THE SOIL ASSOCIATION)

Your questions answered

What does it really mean to be "organic"? How much does organic farming really differ from conventional methods? How worldwide is this approach? Here are some clear answers to common questions.

What does "organic" actually mean?

Organic farmers are those who farm according to organic principles (*see page 244*). They are inspected and certified annually by an approved certification body such as Farm Verified Organic. Organic foods, drinks, and goods are produced from certified organic crops and ingredients. By law, *only* certified foods or goods can be sold as "organic".

Do organic standards vary from country to country?

Yes. Different countries have different growing conditions and practices that must be taken into account. However, all standards must conform to basic legal requirements, as laid down in statutory regulations such as those of the European Union. Some certifying bodies, such as the Soil Association, in the UK, may set additional standards above the legal minimum required.

Do organic farmers use pesticides?

A small number of predominantly natural pesticides are allowed in certain circumstances. Because all pesticides – whether natural or synthetic – are harmful, organic farmers must often seek written consent from their certifying body before using them. All permitted pesticides are subject to constant review and will be removed from the permitted list as soon as better natural controls are developed.

Are antibiotics banned from organic farms?

No. Conventional medication – including antibiotics – must always be and is always given where it is necessary to prevent suffering. On organic farms animals are treated on an individual basis, however, and the withdrawal time before the animal can then be sold is at least twice as long (or even three times as long under certain rules) as the withdrawal times for conventionally raised animals.

Are organic yields always lower and, if so, why?

Organic farmers operate extensive systems, which means they keep fewer animals on a given area, and some of the available land is used to build up natural fertility, for example by growing green manures that cannot be used for grazing or sold as a crop. During the conversion period, withdrawal of artificial fertilizers and pesticides can also cause reduced yields initially. Once established, however, organic farms are highly productive and yields match or sometimes even exceed conventional equivalents.

Is organic as economical as conventional?

Organic farming is very cost effective and represents the true cost of producing high-quality food and other goods. Organic farms also use less net energy than conventional farms, which rely heavily on external inputs. Unfortunately, the hidden costs of conventional agriculture – pollution, environmental damage, soil erosion, and damage to human health – are not taken into account. Farming subsidies favor intensive systems, distorting further the economics of organic production.

Do organic farmers use only traditional methods?

No. Organic farming uses the best of the old with the best of the new and is constantly refining and developing new sustainable agricultural solutions that will be of long-lasting benefit to farming and to the environment.

Are all organic farms 100 percent organic?

Not necessarily. Farms can convert progressively, if they wish. Because of the shortage of organic feedstuffs, manure, and straw, conventional straw and composted manures from non-intensive farms are allowed, as are a small proportion of approved non-GM feedstuffs. This is a temporary measure, known as a "derogation", and is strictly controlled.

What does "biodynamic" farming mean?

This specialized organic approach to farming and gardening, founded in 1924, treats every farm and garden as unique and self-sustaining, in balance with soil, plant, animal, and cosmic processes, and operates worldwide. Biodynamic farmers and gardeners use special sprays and compost preparations that act as catalysts, and a lunar calendar to determine when to sow and harvest. Their goods will be labeld accordingly.

Can organic farming feed the world?

We already have enough food to feed the world. The reasons so many go hungry are poverty, the politics of distribution, and a global economic framework that considers growing for profit more important than feeding people. Considering the massive environmental problems caused by conventional agriculture, organic farming is the only system which is ever likely to feed and sustain the world in the long term.

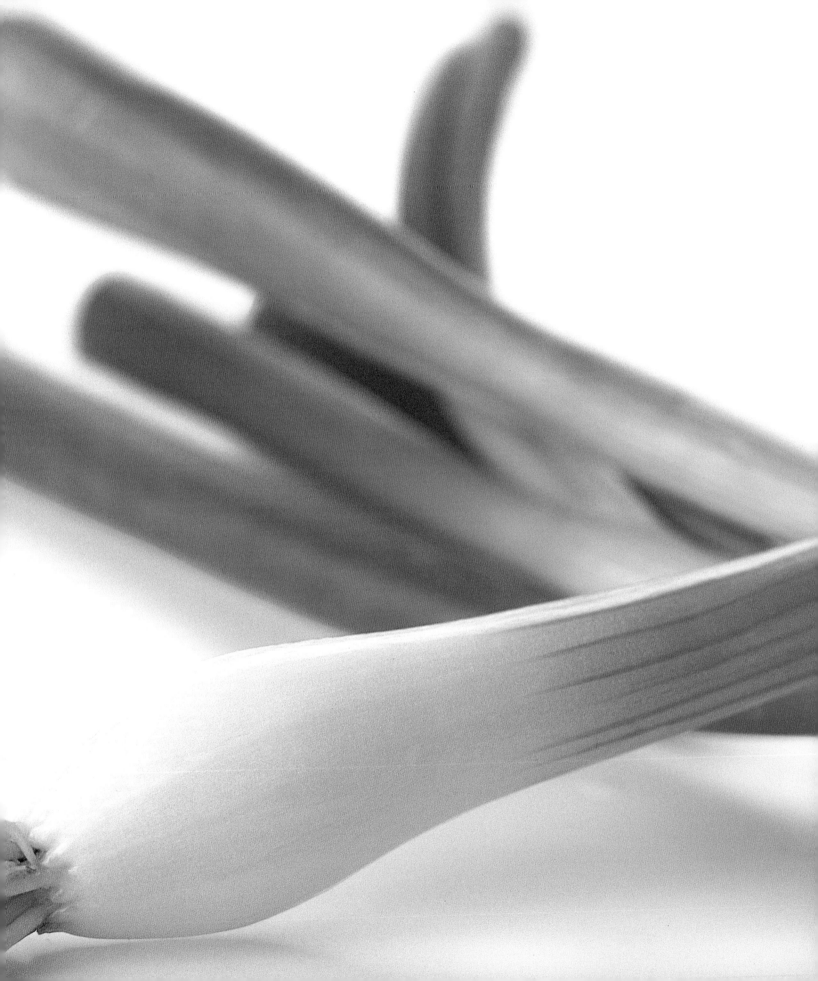

organic
FOOD & DRINK

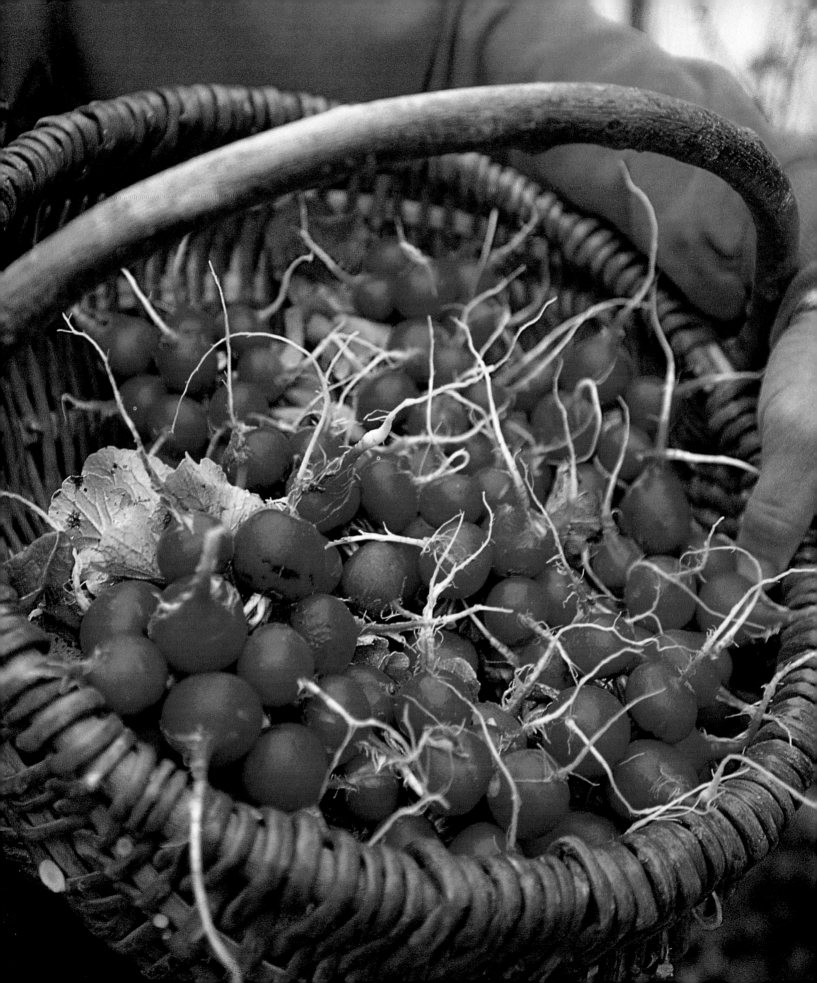

WHY EAT organic

The first step to an eco-lifestyle is to start enjoying some of the huge variety of organic foods you can now buy. In doing so you are choosing the healthiest option for you, your family, and the environment.

Like organic farming, organic food offers you so much more than just food grown without artificial pesticides or fertilizers and animals not raised in intensive conditions or propped up with antibiotics. You will also find that when you switch to organic produce you will start to discover more about how your food is produced and the people who produce and sell it, which will add to your cooking and eating pleasure.

As you begin to realize what eating organic can offer, you will become increasingly aware of the welfare and environmental issues surrounding modern food production. Not many people, for example, automatically think of buying organic bananas or coffee, but read the profiles (*see pages 68 and 104*) and you, too, will be converted. As well as feeling a sense of well-being and pride through choosing organic, you will help to make things better for all of us and our environment. It was not so long ago that organic food was dismissed as a niche – and therefore exclusive –

market. All that has changed. Today organic food is mainstream and available in every major supermarket. There is so much variety, and organic food is so widely available, that there is something to suit everyone. And do not presume that organic food is expensive – you will always find items that match your budget.

GETTING STARTED

You do not need to switch to a totally organic diet to begin enjoying its fruits. Whether you start with a loaf of organic bread from the supermarket or a bunch of freshly harvested organic carrots from a farmer's market, the same positive action will generate the same positive feelings. Many people comment on the flavor of organic food and, once you begin eating it on a regular basis, you will want to adapt your diet, shopping habits, and budget to enable you to choose as much as possible. This section explains everything you need to know to get you started.

Buy at least one organic item every time you shop

Start with everyday staples like bread, milk, potatoes, and pasta

Try something new every week

Snap up promotional and seasonal offers

Go local for best value by joining a boxed food program or visiting a farmer's market

Your questions answered

Why should you try to include organic food in your diet? What does the term "organic food" really mean? Here are answers to some of your most common questions.

What are organic foods?

Organic foods are those that have been produced according to organic farming and processing standards. Only foods and drinks made from ingredients that have been certified as organic can legally be labeled and sold as organic. More on specific standards is included throughout the food and drink section *(see pages 44–113)* and Standards Count *(see page 246)* features general information on classification.

Do organic foods taste better than nonorganic?

Because organic foods are grown naturally and not forced, generally speaking they are likely to have a better flavor than their nonorganic equivalents. Numerous taste tests confirm this, as do the thousands of people who regularly eat organic foods. However, because taste is a personal thing, and depends on a range of factors, a better taste cannot be guaranteed.

How can I be sure foods are genuinely organic?

Wherever they have been produced, all organic foods come with full farm-to-table traceability back to their original source, and every producer or supplier is legally required to provide proof of authenticity. The certification number or label on the package *(see page 246)* is the consumer's guarantee of authenticity. For fresh foods that are sold loose, the producer or supplier will be able to provide proof if asked.

Do organic foods last as long as nonorganic?

This varies. Because no post-harvest chemicals are used, some organic fresh produce does not last as long as nonorganic, but often its lower water content and its nonforced growth mean it may actually last longer. Foods such as sausages and chilled goods contain no artificial preservatives and should be enjoyed as soon as possible. Manufactured organic foods have a shelf life similar to their nonorganic equivalents.

Why are organic foods potentially healthier?

Organic foods are foods you can trust and feel good about, and eating them brings many benefits. Uniquely, they contain no hydrogenated fats, artificial additives, flavorings, or preservatives, as well as being produced without the use of artificial pesticides, genetically modified organisms (GMOs), or routine antibiotics. In addition, organic fresh produce generally has lower nitrate levels and can have higher mineral and vitamin C content *(see page 26)*.

What about the cost?

Organic foods represent the true cost of growing nutritious, high-quality produce. Foods grown using modern intensive methods may be cheap, but have very high health, social, and environmental costs, like that of cleaning up water pollution. Unfortunately, organic foods are often unfairly judged against mass-produced foods, which distorts the value for money ratio. However, the increasing production and availability of organic foods is rapidly making them more affordable.

Do organic foods contain any additives?

Organic foods are processed with the minimum processing necessary for each type of foodstuff. A limited number of natural processing aids *(see page 245)*, such as ascorbic acid (vitamin C) or guar gum, are approved and will be clearly labeled on the packaging. All are under constant review and no new processing aid is added without the closest scrutiny.

Are organic manufactured foods entirely organic?

The vast majority of organic foods on sale are 100 percent organic. However, standards allow for a small proportion of some nonorganic ingredients to be used temporarily, in certain circumstances *(see page 244)*. Any nonorganic ingredient will be clearly labeled as such on the packaging.

Are organic foods pesticide-free?

Because pesticides are endemic – in the air, the ground, and the water supplies – and therefore the risk of contamination is always present, it is impossible for organic farming to claim to be entirely pesticide-free. Since organic foods are produced without the use of artificial pesticides, however, direct exposure to pesticide residues in organic foods is effectively reduced to zero.

What about GM foods?

Organic standards exclude genetically modified organisms (GMOs) of any kind from the growing, processing or manufacture of organic foods. This ban includes all derivatives as well as the GM enzymes used to make rennet for vegetarian cheese. Many organic manufacturers also test their products independently to ensure GM purity.

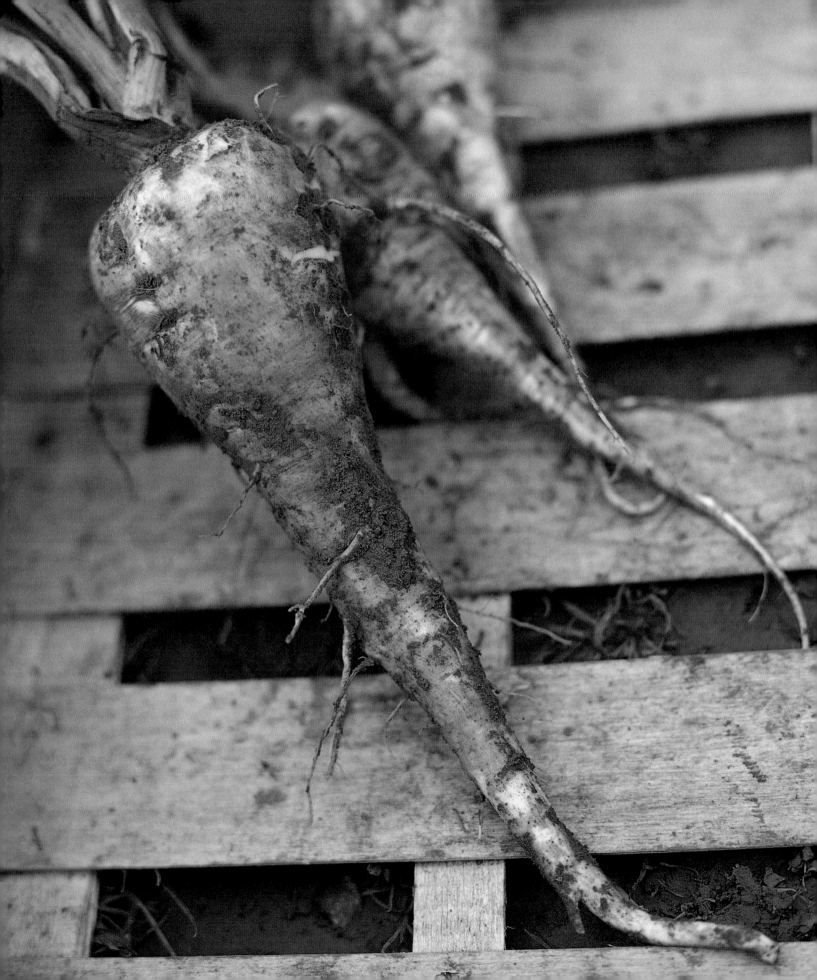

Fresh is best

Good health begins with including as much wholesome fresh produce as possible in our daily diet. Nutritionists recommend that we eat at least five portions of fresh fruit and vegetables every day.

Fresh produce is central to a healthy diet and for most people this now means choosing organic whenever possible. Happily, production of organic fresh produce is rising exponentially worldwide, which means that availability has improved enormously. Major retailers stock organic fruit and vegetables, as do many independent shops and smaller chains. Organic supermarkets have the largest selection, while local organic boxed food plans offer the best value. If you have a garden, the ideal solution, of course, is to grow your own (*see page 168*).

AVAILABILITY

Because it is grown naturally, there is more seasonal variation in organic produce than in conventional. Also, since some crops grow better organically in some countries than others, imported organic produce will always play an important role and help make up any shortfall. However, unlike conventional crops, organic crops always benefit the local people and local environment (*see page 38*). In the UK up to 80 percent of fresh produce is imported, more of which could be home-grown. The main obstacle is lack of government support, which means British growers are converting more slowly than those in countries where government support is strong.

FOR APPEARANCE'S SAKE

Organic produce is not uniform, but is a celebration of nature's individuality. Nor is cosmetic perfection desirable (up to 80 percent of pesticides are said to be used to ensure blemish-free crops). This means there is a greater variability in size and shape in organic fruit and vegetables and sometimes more surface blemishes. Generally, too, you can expect two main differences in the eating quality of organic and nonorganic produce: a greater intensity and sweetness, and more texture. Organic beauty is thus more than skin-deep and it is health and taste that matter most.

ORGANIC STANDARDS

All fresh vegetables and fruit labeled "organic" must, by law, be grown according to the following standards:

✤ Crops are grown without the use of artificial fertilizers or pesticides
✤ Generally, the required conversion period to organic methods is two years (for ground crops) or three years (for perennials)
✤ Appropriate crop rotation is practiced for ground crops to break pest and disease cycles, and to help maintain soil fertility and structure
✤ No post-harvest chemical treatments are used
✤ Fertility is provided by natural organic manures, composts and fertilizers
✤ No use of GM seeds or other materials is permitted

A taste of summer

Blue skies and sunny days bring forth a wealth of variety of good things to eat. Fresh organic summer produce is packed with natural goodness, is quick to prepare and a joy to eat.

Whether you buy them straight from the farm gate, through a boxed food plan, or at the supermarket, the great variety of organic summer vegetables means there is something for everyone.

summer roots

Seasonal bunches of organic turnips, radishes, beets, and summer carrots are a delight. Very often they come with their leaves attached – an extra bonus. No need to peel, just washing with a brush. For added eye appeal, do not cut off the whiskery roots of baby root vegetables. Local boxed food producers often grow yellow and striped varieties of organic beets, as well as kohlrabi. Baby beet leaves are as tender as spinach and can be eaten raw, as in salads, or cooked.

Cook's tip Cook baby carrots and turnips in butter with a few chopped herbs. A pinch of organic sugar also brings out their sweetness.

lettuce

Organic lettuces have more heart and soul than most conventional lettuces, and are closer in taste and texture to home-grown lettuces. The majority of conventionally grown lettuces are cultivated by highly intensive methods, often hydroponically. Organic lettuces are always grown in soil; they are allowed to grow at a natural rate and have natural resilience. In summer, locally grown organic lettuce is easy to come by. If buying from a local grower you may need to discard the outer leaves, and watch out for the occasional friendly insect or slug. Imported organic lettuces from other countries are available most of the year. Popular organic varieties are Little Gem and the various red and green frilly varieties such as red leaf and green leaf.

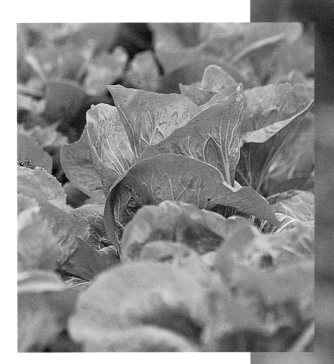

Prepackaged organic salad packs are also becoming popular. Unlike many conventional packaged salads, they are not washed in chlorine. They may be washed with very dilute solutions of citric acid to help keep them fresh, but this does not affect the flavor. In summer you can grow organic lettuces for yourself very easily (*see page 170*).

Cook's tip Stew the shredded outer leaves in butter *à la française*, with organic peas and finely chopped carrots and onions, for a side dish.

tomatoes

Conventional greenhouse tomatoes are grown using biological controls instead of artificial pesticides these days, but only organic tomatoes are all cultivated in soil and fed naturally. In summer

tomatoes are available locally grown or you can grow them yourself. In winter they are usually shipped from California and other warmer climes. The riper the tomatoes are, the better the flavor, and, at their best, organic tomatoes have a firm texture and a sweet, intense flavor. Cherry tomatoes are naturally sweeter than other types and have the highest vitamin C content.

Cook's tip If unripe, leave tomatoes for a few days at room temperature to develop their flavor. Unless very ripe, never keep tomatoes in the refrigerator.

peas & beans

Organic producers cultivate a wide variety of peas and beans, ranging from sugar snap peas, snow peas, lima beans and yellow, purple, and green French

A taste of summer

beans all the way through to drying beans such as borlotti beans, which are all available seasonally. Organic French beans, sugar snap peas, and snow peas, both locally grown and imported, are now available throughout most of the year. Organic peas are full of flavor but, because they are grown naturally, they do not necessarily all ripen at the same time, and this can cause variations in tenderness.

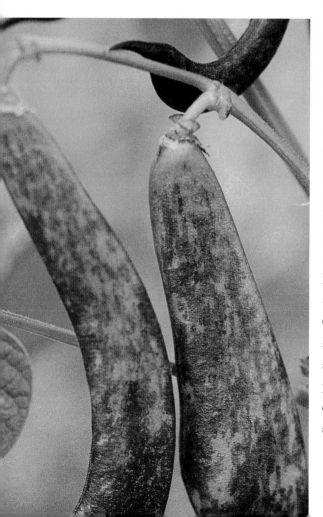

Cook's tip Do not undercook French beans – they are best when just soft. They are delicious served as a salad, tossed in a dressing made from olive oil mixed with toasted, ground organic hazelnuts, and seasoned with salt.

broccoli & cauliflower

Organic broccoli has real flavor and vibrancy while organic cauliflower has beautifully creamy curds with extra flavor to match. Broccoli is known as a "superfood" and a powerful antioxidant. Both are available for most of the year, either grown in the US or imported. Other than a careful check for insects in the folds of the curds, they need no preparation, except dividing into florets. Store both in the salad drawer of the refrigerator. They are best eaten as soon as possible, although freshly harvested cauliflower will keep in good condition stored cold for up to a week.
Cook's tip Both broccoli and cauliflower are best cooked briefly until just soft, and make excellent salads, including pasta salads. Broccoli stalks are good to eat – peel off the outer stems then chop and cook as usual.

spinach

A recent research study found organic spinach samples to have almost 100 percent more iron and manganese than conventional samples. Like other organic green leafy produce, it is also lower in nitrates. So choose organic spinach when you can. It does not store well and should be eaten as soon as possible. Wash the leaves well just before cooking.
Cook's tip Stir-fry, or blanch briefly in a pan of water, gently squeezing out the excess water. For extra tenderness remove the stems from large leaves first.

fennel

Fennel produced organically has a powerful flavor and is extra-crunchy. It will often be misshapen, and its outer leaves may be slightly tough – use these for soups and stocks. Locally grown organic fennel is available in the US from summer to late autumn, but organic fennel, imported from warmer climates, is available for most of the year.
Cook's tip For the best summer salad, slice fennel thinly and dress with olive oil and finely chopped tarragon or olives. In autumn combine with finely sliced organic oranges.

eggplants & peppers

Organic peppers and eggplants are becoming commonplace. A range of varieties is cultivated by local growers, often for boxed food plans, but for the retail market they might be imported. Peppers will ripen naturally and further develop their flavor, so store at room temperature and not in the refrigerator. Both are superb cooked on the barbecue and can be grown at home in pots.

Cook's tip Modern eggplant varieties do not need to be salted first, although this will prevent them from soaking up as much olive oil as they might otherwise during the cooking process.

avocados

Delicious, highly nutritious, and rich in vitamin E and essential fatty acids, organic avocados are a popular choice and many growers in California and Mexico are converting to organic methods. The main varieties are Hass and Fuerte, which are both readily available in the US for most of the year. Perfect for salsas, instant dips, salads, lunches, and dinners, these offer good all around value – no organic home should be without them.

Cook's tip Ripe, soft avocados should be eaten as soon as possible, but will last for two to three days in the refrigerator.

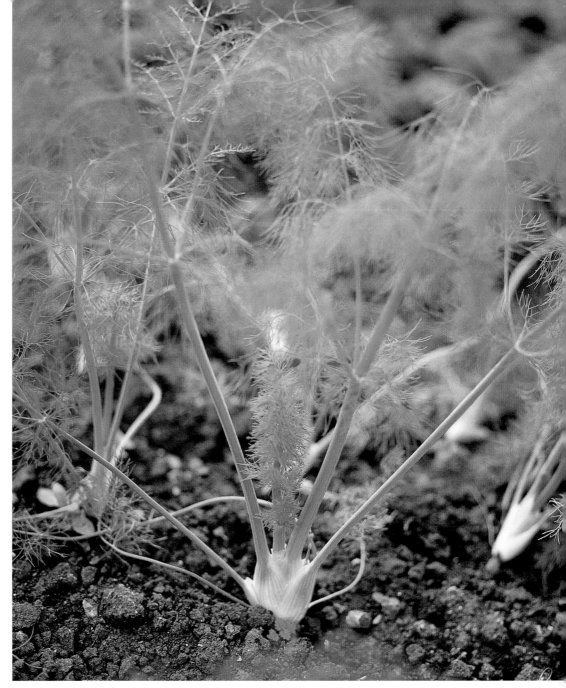

garlic

Fresh summer garlic is much easier on the digestion than the dried version, and is wonderful roasted or puréed. Local growers offer freshly harvested organic garlic in summer – perfect for barbecues, pesto, and garlic mayonnaise (aïoli). Organic garlic is is often grown locally but is also shipped from other states year- round. You can easily grow garlic organically at home (*see page 171*).

Cook's tip Garlic should be kept cool at all times. Sprouting cloves are not good to eat, but they can be planted in a pot or in the ground and the garlic-flavored shoots used as a springtime herb.

Focus on corn

Organic corn – corn on the cob – is a real treat, with a rich flavor and natural creamy sweetness. Summer barbecues would not be the same without it. Organic corn, or maize, meanwhile, is a golden treasure in a world increasingly threatened by genetic modification.

Originating in Central and South America, corn is one of the earliest known domestic crops and has been in cultivation for thousands of years. Modern varieties are usually yellow, but traditional varieties (*see below right*) come in a range of colors, from orange, red, and brown to a deep purple-blue or black. Starchy varieties, used for flour, polenta, popcorn, corn breads, tortillas, cornflakes, and animal feed, are known as maize, while sweet varieties are known just as corn.

big business

In the US, maize is a major commodity crop, grown as intensively as wheat and used extensively in animal feeds and in processed foods. The eco-facts are:

❖ In 1945 no insecticides were used on maize, which was grown in rotation with other crops. Today, half the maize grown is cultivated as a monocrop and the use of insecticides has increased 1,000-fold.

❖ In 1945 the corn rootworm pest was not a problem. Since using pesticides, crop losses from this pest have risen from 3½ percent to 12 percent.

❖ About a third of the maize grown in the US is genetically engineered to contain *bacillus thuringiensis* (Bt), a soil bacterium used by organic growers to control caterpillars and other pests. Cultivation of the genetically modified (GM) maize will inevitably cause insect resistance to Bt over time, robbing organic growers of one of their most valuable natural insecticides. In an attempt to stop the rapid development of the resistance that is already building up, conventional maize farmers in Mississippi are prohibited from growing more than half their crop with Bt maize.

the GM threat

GM maize is already widely grown in the US (*see right*). Because it can cross-pollinate with non-GM corn varieties,

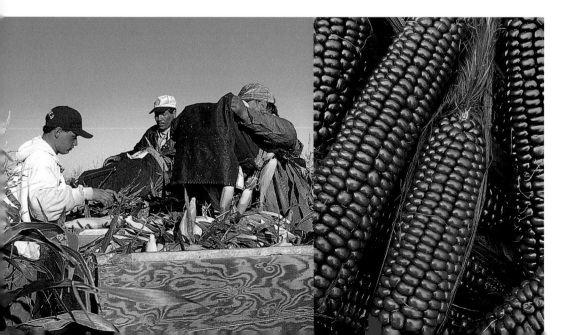

including corn, this has created an important precedent in the fight to be GM-free. Research has confirmed that pollen travels much further than previously thought. This means that, under current regulations, GM maize field trials in the UK and the rest of Europe pose a threat to the purity of all organic and non-GM corn. Riverford Farm in Devon, which runs one of the UK's most successful organic boxed food plans, is a case in point. In 1999 12 acres of its organic corn were threatened with contamination from nearby GM maize trials, and the grower was in danger of losing his organic status for his crop. Increasingly this is happening to other organic farmers too. In the case of the UK, the Soil Association is campaigning for all growers of non-GM varieties of corn to be properly protected from GM contamination. Buying organic and choosing not to buy processed foods containing conventional corn ingredients is the best way of ensuring our organic corn remains GM-free.

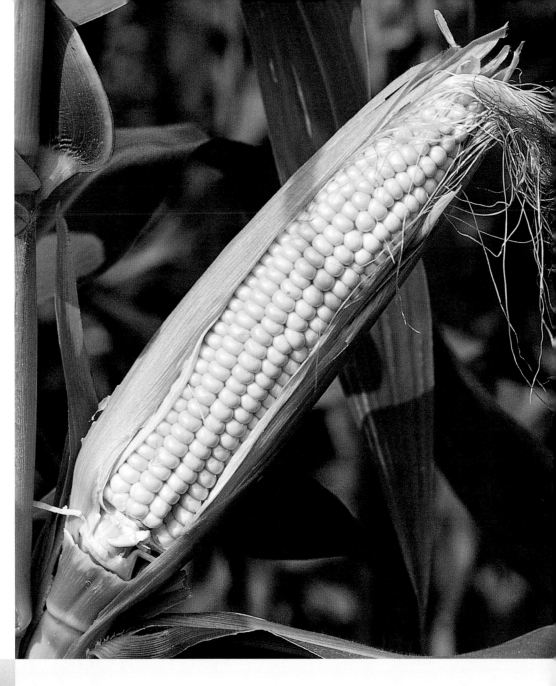

NATURE'S WAY

Organic corn is nature's sunshine in a cob. Herbicides are forbidden, so organic growers will hand-weed, or use weed-brushing machines until the crop is growing well. In the UK pests are not generally a major problem. The ripe cobs are picked by hand and the stubbles are ploughed back into the soil where they rot down to provide organic matter. Corn is a seasonal crop available from mid- to late summer. It is usually sold with its leaves and brown "tassle", and is a favorite vegetable at farmer's markets all over the country.

Cook's tip Tender corn will exude a milky liquid when the kernel is pressed between your finger and thumbnail. It is best cooked as soon as possible, but also freezes very well.

A winter wonderland

There are few better ways to brighten those cold winter months than by enjoying the depth of flavor and healthy boost you can get from organic winter vegetables – the ultimate comfort foods.

The ever-increasing range of organic winter vegetables now available, both imported and home-grown, means that it has never been easier to choose organic, whatever the season.

celery

Organic celery has good flavor and a loud crunch. It is perfect for crudités and is one of the best vegetables for adding flavor to casseroles and salads. Widely grown in the US, it is also imported. Fresh American home-grown organic is best, especially the deep green varieties, which have a superb flavor, although the outside stalks may be tougher. Celery stores well for up to two weeks in the refrigerator.

Cook's tip Use the outside leaves and stalks for juicing, or in soups and stocks. Scatter the tender inner leaves, finely chopped, over salads and pork dishes.

winter roots

Taste freshly dug organic carrots, parsnips, beets, or celeriac and you will rediscover the true earthy sweetness of root vegetables. Carrots are the most popular organic vegetable and locally grown carrots can usually be found in supermarkets or farmer's markets, all year round. Unwashed roots last better than washed ones and all should be stored dry, in the dark, or in the refrigerator, and removed from any plastic bags first.

Cook's tip Finely grating root vegetables brings out their sweetness. To make an instant healthly winter salad, grate whatever mixture of roots you like, along with a small apple if you wish. Dress with an olive oil and lemon vinaigrette or some mayonnaise and serve as a side salad.

leeks

One of the best winter vegetables, organic leeks often come with more green flag (leaves) and, if freshly dug, will probably need careful washing. They are available from early autumn onwards. The outer tough green flags on leeks should be discarded, but the

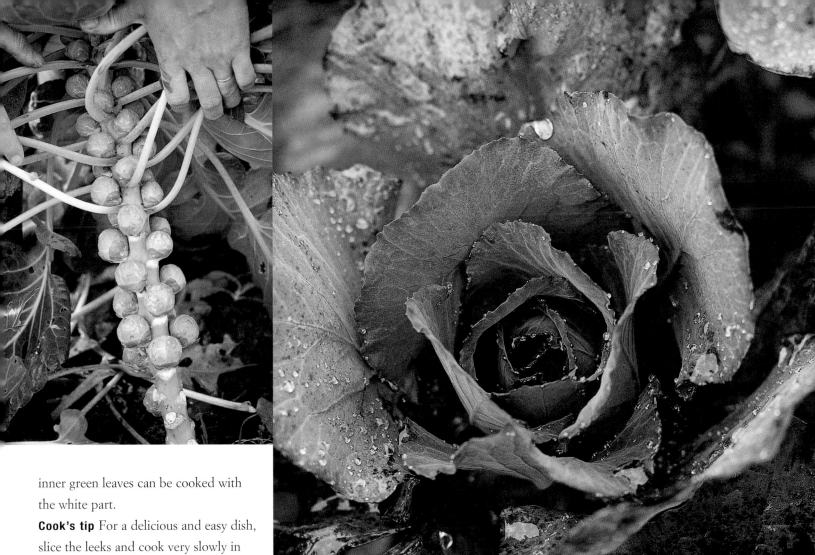

inner green leaves can be cooked with the white part.

Cook's tip For a delicious and easy dish, slice the leeks and cook very slowly in organic olive oil with chopped organic red pepper for 40 minutes, or until meltingly soft, adding a little chopped rosemary if you wish.

dark greens

These include organic cabbages, purple and white sprouting broccoli, Brussels sprouts, spring greens, Swiss chard, spinach beet, and vivid green and purple kales. When freshly harvested, all are generally superb. All, too, contain fistfuls of vitamins and antioxidants. Always a favorite gardener's vegetable, and popular on here in the US, thanks to

farmer's markets, organic Swiss chard is becoming more common in the US and may soon appear in supermarkets. Organic Brussels sprouts often come attached to their stalks – a sure sign of freshness. Organic cabbages will store well for a week or so in the refrigerator. Other greens should be eaten in their prime. You may well find the occasional insect lurking within, so remember

to check them carefully.

Cook's tip All greens should be cooked either very quickly – shredding and stir-frying is fast and easy – or long and slowly. For something different, briefly blanch Swiss chard or any kind of broccoli, drain, then cook very slowly in olive oil, chili, and garlic. Season with salt, drizzle with extra olive oil, and eat as a side dish.

A winter
wonderland

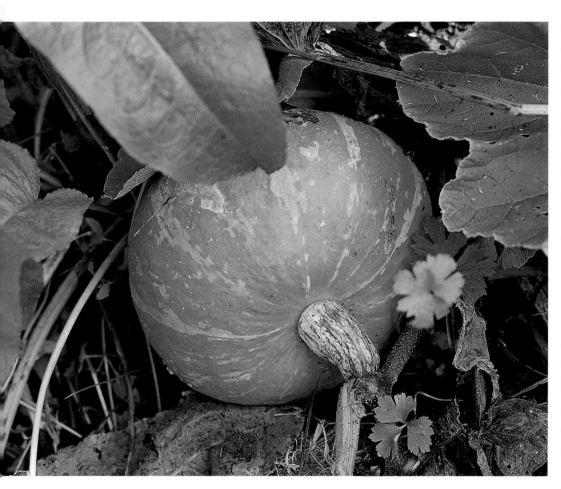

smooth texture, are highly nutritious, and are easily digestible too. The orange-fleshed varieties such as Dumpling and Acorn are the best. Organic squash is easy to grow at home and is a common sight at farmer's markets. Some varieties may also be available in supermarkets. **Cook's tip** Squash make superlative soups and purées and are excellent when cut into wedges, brushed with olive oil, and simply roasted.

sprouting seeds

These are one of the healthiest and easiest ways to add vitamins to your winter salads. Look out for organic beansprouts, alfalfa, chickpeas, and mixed bean sprouts in the refrigerated aisle of the supermarket. Always use them as soon as possible.

mushrooms

The development of organic cultivated mushrooms has been a great success, though changes to European Union regulations may mean Europeans will soon have fewer available. At the moment, they are an organic stalwart, readily available all year round, and a good first choice for everyone. Varieties

chinese leaves

Farmer's markets often have a large assortment of peppery Chinese leafy vegetables such as mizuna, bok choi, mustard, komatsuna, and chrysanthemum greens. Examine the leaves and use as soon as possible. Small, tender leaves are good for salads; otherwise, shred

and stir-fry for a couple of minutes with ginger, garlic, and soy sauce, or with a sweet-and-sour Chinese sauce.

squash

Squash are the winter vegetable par excellence. They store well until spring, have a rich, satisfying flavor, a dense,

include organic brown caps, buttons, creminis, and shiitake (grown on logs). Except for the latter, they are cultivated naturally on composted straw in specialized mushroom sheds and take five to six weeks to grow. Cultivating mushrooms organically requires the highest standards (*see below*), with the spent compost being recycled for use as a soil conditioner and fertilizer.

Cook's tip Mushrooms need to breathe and quickly deteriorate when stored in plastic wrap or bags. Take them out of their wrapping and store in a brown paper bag in the refrigerator or loose on a plate lined with paper towels.

THE DIFFERENCES THAT COUNT

✤ In organic mushroom production there is a total absence of the many different types of chemicals that are approved for use in conventional mushroom-growing sheds

✤ Up to four times as many people are employed to monitor organic mushrooms

✤ Any sign of disease is removed by hand

✤ Only biodegradable disinfectants are used to clean the sheds between crops

watercress

Organic watercress is a winter "superfood" that packs a healthy punch. Traditional British grower John Hurd's organic watercress is grown completely naturally and cut by hand, and is widely available from March to December in British supermarkets and organic shops.

Cook's tip Watercress lasts only two to three days, and is best kept boxed in the refrigerator. Pick it over carefully. Chopped watercress adds a peppery kick to salads, salsas, or pestos, and is good scattered over fish or chicken dishes.

potatoes

Taste tests consistently show that many people find organic potatoes to be superior in flavor. If you eat the skins, always choose organic, since these are not sprayed with any post-harvest insecticides or sprout suppressants – although remember that this means that the potatoes will not keep as long. Organic potatoes are easy to find. Popular commercial varieties include Yukon Gold, red, and fingerlings. Local growers and farmer's markets often sell traditional and heritage varieties. Organic potatoes are grown in Germany, Holland, Austria, Spain, and France, and organic new potatoes in Egypt, Israel, Italy, and Morocco.

Cook's tip Potatoes must be stored properly – thick brown paper bags are best – and kept in the dark at all times.

preprepared vegetables

Pre-cut organic vegetables, such as broccoli spears and runner beans, are becoming available in supermarkets. As with packaged salad, washing in

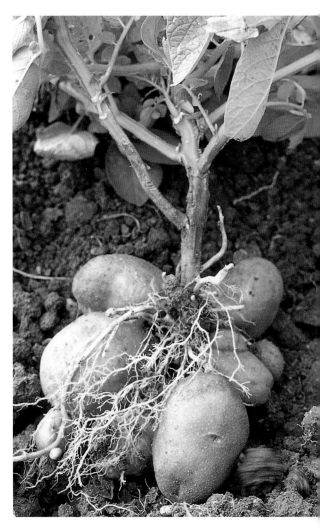

chlorine solutions is forbidden (*see page 53*). Frozen organic vegetables (*see page 98*) are also available from supermarkets and organic shops.

winter salads

Salad leaves provide a bright note and are as important for health in winter as in summer. Farmer's markets often carry a selection of leaves, including a wide variety of multi-colored, slightly bitter-tasting chicories.

Power plants

Organic herbs and spices are a "must" for all your cooking. They are available both fresh and dried and can be relied on for their quality and purity.

Organic herbs and spices are neither grown with artificial nutrients or pesticides nor allowed to be irradiated. They are a high-value, labor-intensive crop sourced worldwide from over 30 countries, including Madagascar, the US, Egypt, Sri Lanka, Uganda, Turkey, Hungary, Indonesia, Spain, and Pakistan. The industry is small and personal, with growers, specialist importers, and experts working closely together to ensure the highest standards.

herb gardens

In the US fresh culinary organic herbs are now available most of the year. Local growers often sell by the bunch at farmer's markets; otherwise they are shipped from other locations. There are several brands of dried organic herbs and spices to choose from. All have either been grown to organic standards or are "wild-crafted", which means they have been harvested from isolated places under strict regulations that ensure purity and the preservation of the natural habitat. One organic expert, Hambleden Herbs, based in Somerset, is Britain's leading organic herb and spice company. It sources worldwide and offers more than 500 organic herb and spice products, including herbal teas, infusions, culinary herbs, and mulling spices. It has its own drying barn and also grows 100 varieties of medicinal herbs (*see left*) from which it produces its own fresh herbal tinctures made on the farm.

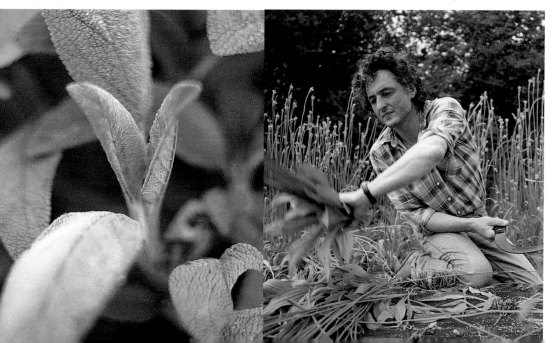

The devil's claw project is now providing a fairly traded, stable income for some of Namibia's poorest rural communities.

CYRIL LOMBARD, CENTRE FOR RESEARCH, INFORMATION & ACTION IN AFRICA

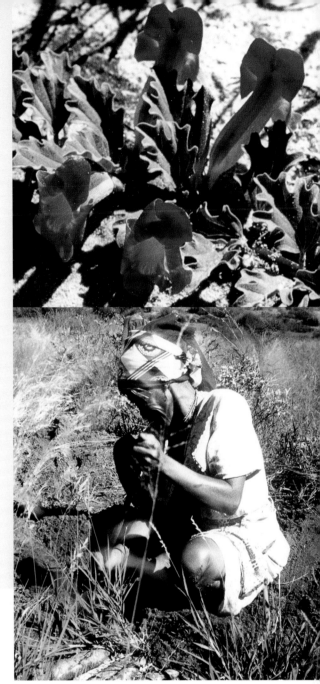

AFRICAN INITIATIVES

Exciting organic initiatives are taking place in Africa, where organic herbs and spices are providing valuable jobs and income as well as developing new, sustainable agricultural practices and helping to revitalize rural economies in countries such as Malawi, Zambia, and Namibia.

FARMING DEVIL'S CLAW

In a ground-breaking initiative, more than 740,000 acres of semi-desert in Namibia were recently certified organic for the sustainable harvesting of devil's claw root (*see right*), which is used to make a valuable herbal remedy for arthritis. The project is funded by local and international agencies and has resulted in increased prices for the harvesters who receive the proper training in managing their resource. As a result, the quality of the devil's claw now being harvested has also improved. The project is now providing a fairly traded stable income for some of the country's poorest rural communities, who now trade directly with the exporters. The exporters also contribute to a community-controlled fund that is helping to develop other community benefits.

the producers

fresh or dried

For maximum flavor it is important that herbs and spices are dried in carefully controlled conditions.

If dried too quickly they may have a bright color but will have lost much of their volatile oils, which means their flavor can suffer. If dried too slowly, they will not store well. Like conventional varieties, organic dried herbs and spices last for between 18 months and two years. Once opened, ground spices and powdered herbs gradually lose their potency and, if possible, should be used within three to six months. Fresh herbs with fragile leaves such as dill, chervil, basil, and fennel should be used as soon as possible, preferably within two days. Other fresh herbs such as parsley, cilantro, and chives will last up to one week. Tough-leaved herbs such as oregano, thyme, sage, rosemary, and bay leaves will dry naturally in the kitchen and do not need to be stored in the refrigerator.

Pick of the crops

Fruit should be enjoyed as nature intended. Currently, organic fruit is only being produced on a small scale, making every fruit available an even more precious gift.

Organic fruit is enjoyed in varying degrees around the world. Dependable climates, such as those in sunny, dry countries, produce more organic fruit. This makes home-grown organic fruit a real treat in areas that do not produce much of their own and is why most of the organic fruit bought in those countries is imported.

berries

Organic berries are seasonal delights, full of sunshine and nature's vitamins. Although supply is limited, supermarkets regularly stock seasonal organic strawberries, raspberries, and blueberries, and have organic cranberries at Christmas (*see page 36*). Local farmer's markets often sell varieties such as black-, red-,

and whitecurrants, hybrid berries such as loganberries, and large, fat, juicy cultivated blackberries. Organic growers tend to grow a wider range of varieties, choosing those that are most suited to their conditions. Although, in some ways, they are not as challenging as organic tree fruits to grow, organic berry fruits are much more fragile. Nature intended for them to be eaten as soon after harvesting as possible, and because the fruit is not force-fed, the flavor is generally excellent, and can be truly superb. Currently, only a handful of growers, in the UK for example, are producing organic strawberries commercially, with most appearing as summer treats at farmer's markets. Imported strawberries tend to come mostly from South America.

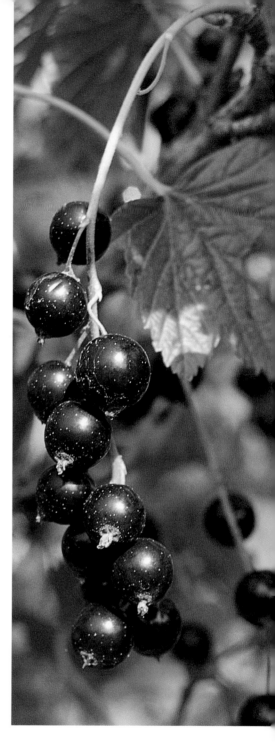

THE DIFFERENCES THAT COUNT

❖ Organic strawberry growers in the US choose varieties with resistance to mildew, such as Florence and Pegasus. The most common strawberry is Elsanta, which gives high yields but is prone to disease and needs regular spraying.

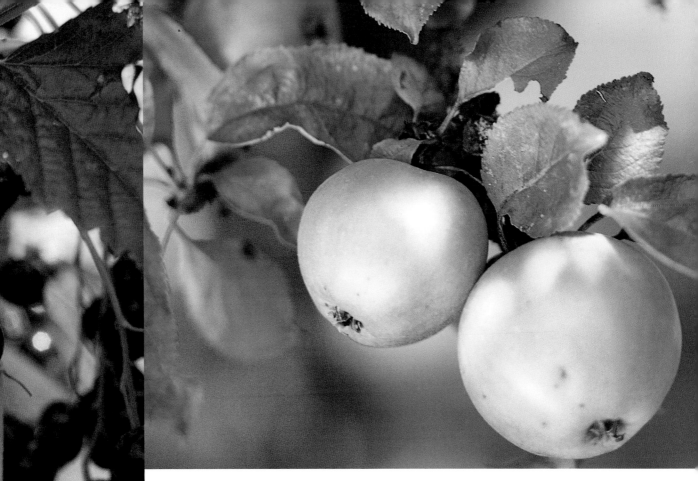

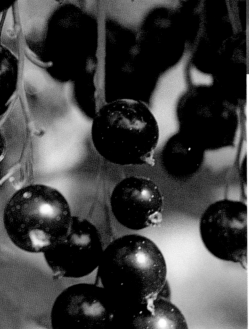

of the land, while most growers feed their crops with artificial fertilizers.

✤ The fungicide methyl bromide is forbidden in organic strawberry production. Methyl bromide is banned in several countries as a class 1 ozone-depleter but is still permitted in the UK and is not expected to be phased out there until 2010.

Cook's tip For an instant *petit four*, dip perfect strawberries (with the stalks on) into a little melted organic dark chocolate and let set. The remainder of the strawberries can be used to make cooling summer soups and refreshing drinks, milkshakes, smoothies, ices, and sorbets.

apples & pears

Grown in many countries, including the US, Canada, Argentina, Chile, and several European countries, apples and pears are the most readily available organic fruits. Rather than maximizing yields, organic growers concentrate on building up the health of their orchards by providing fertility programs, encouraging natural predators and maximum biodiversity and using

✤ Organic strawberries are planted up to 20 percent further apart than the majority of strawberries, to allow for adequate ventilation.

✤ Organic strawberries are grown in rotation with other crops and derive nourishment from the natural fertility

Pick of the crops

seaweed-based foliar sprays. The result is fruit with real character and often thicker, protective skins. As American growers understand only too well, without a cushion of pesticides, blemishes are inevitable. Without artificial fertilizers to make the trees produce high yields and large fruits, volumes are smaller. Together with the extra time, effort and manpower involved in growing organically, this means the fruit naturally costs more, but each is as nature intended – unique.

stone fruits

Organic stone fruits, including apricots, peaches, nectarines, and even plums, are in scarcer supply than some exotic fruits.

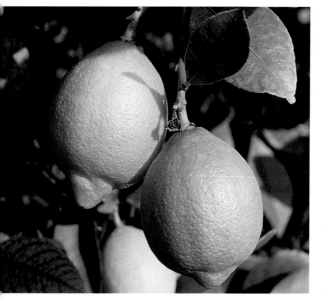

Very few stores sell them, and then only occasionally. This makes them even more precious. They bruise easily, so need extra care. Dried organic apricots and apple slices are readily available. Keep a pack handy in the pantry cupboard (*see page 92*).

citrus fruits

A full range of organic citrus fruit is now available, including grapefruits, oranges, clementines, tangerines, limes, and lemons. Organic juicing oranges are available in bulk. They are not waxed or treated with post-harvest fungicides so, once ripe, store them in the refrigerator.
Cook's tip Organic citrus fruits can be used in many ways – to flavor meat and vegetable dishes, in desserts and drinks, to make candied organic citrus peel, and Moroccan preserved lemons.

exotic fruits

Organic melons, pineapples, mangoes, papaya, and kiwi fruit are year round treats, and are becoming increasingly available in supermarkets. Organic tropical fruit is ususally imported. It comes from all over the world inlcuding South America, the Caribbean, and

Spain. Because of their tough skins, each of these fruits can be stored at room temperature if necessary, to ripen to perfection. Organic kiwi fruit is both exotic and commonplace and has been a major commercial success. The kiwi fruit has a richer flavor when organically grown and is one of the most valuable natural sources of vitamin C. In its natural habitat it is a trailing plant that can live for up to 30 years. Organic kiwi fruits are grown in Italy, France, Chile, and New Zealand. The soil is not sprayed with artificial herbicides and local weed populations are allowed to flourish, helping to keep the soil structure intact and providing a natural habitat for beneficial insects.
Cook's tip Organic pineapples make a perfect ingredient for sweet and savory dishes. Organic melons make cooling summer soups or, when combined with chopped organic strawberries and mint, are the perfect summer first course. Organic kiwi fruits should be eaten when slightly soft. Unless they are already ripe, there is no rush to eat them, since they last well for up to a month, without any loss of vitamin C. To ripen, leave them in a sealed bag with an apple for two to three days.

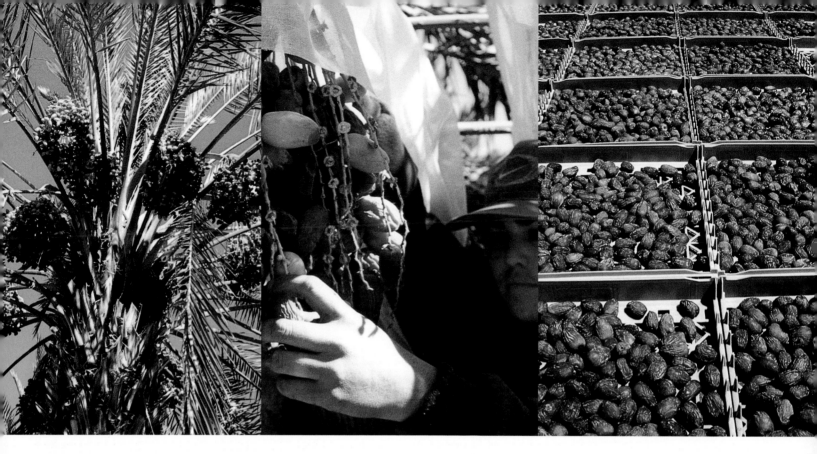

the producers

MAKE IT A DATE

Californian dates are the latest fruit to go organic and are deliciously rich. Few fruits are more ancient or as exotic. At the Oasis Date Gardens in the Coachella Valley (*see above*), the finest date variety for eating fresh – the Medjool, known as the "perfect" date – needs to be treated with great care: hand-thinning, natural ripening, and careful picking by hand ensure a top-quality product.

In California the trees can grow to 70–100 ft (20–30 m) tall. Each acre contains 50 female palms with one male palm to provide the pollen for the female plants. Each year, growers climb the male trees to collect the blossom, before pollinating each female fruit by hand, by attaching a sprig of male blossom to each of the female ones. Unlike many fruits, the dates are allowed to ripen naturally on the trees to ensure maximum sweetness and flavor. This means each tree is picked over three or four times, with the ripest fruit being selected each time. To grow them organically, specially designed bags are placed over the date bunches to protect them from insect attack, and bats and other beneficial natural predators are encouraged to help keep down populations of mosquitos and other pests.

Cook's tip Fresh pitted organic dates make elegant and unusual canapés. Stuff them with organic hummus, crème fraîche, and smoked salmon, or soft cheese flavored with chopped herbs, spice paste, or chopped walnuts.

Demand continues to grow as more people realize the value of eating organic foods.

JIM FREIMUTH, THE OASIS DATE GARDENS

Focus on bananas

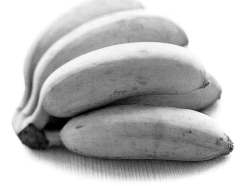

The organic banana is an inspiring example of how organic and fair trade (*see page 220*) principles, together with consumer power, can work to make real changes for the better.

Bananas are one of the most popular fruit in the US, and they are tremendously good for us. Each of us eats around 22 lb (10 kg) of bananas every year, almost all of which, unfortunately, are intensively produced under conditions that have often been heavily criticized. The development of bananas as a major commodity has been – and still remains in many places – a dismal tale of worker and environmental exploitation.

time for change

There are solutions to these problems, however, and with the help of consumers the tide is turning. Buying organic or Fairtrade bananas when you can ensures improved working conditions and health for the workers, and helps to repair and to maintain the environment in which the bananas are grown. It will also send clear messages to major banana companies to

follow the organic and Fairtrade lead and change their production and working practices. Because of consumer pressure, large retailers in the UK, for example, are selling more and more Fairtrade and organic bananas, and demand is rising fast.

plantations

Most organic bananas sold in Europe come from the Dominican Republic, but they are also grown in Israel, Mexico, Martinique, Egypt, Honduras, and Brazil. The banana plant looks like a palm and dies back every year after it has fruited, before growing a new trunk. Managed organically, banana plants are excellent soil-builders. They offer permanent shade and the crop debris builds rich humus. Extra soil fertility is provided by a variety of sources, including animal dung, green manures, coffee husks, guano, fish bones, and seaweed. In some plantations

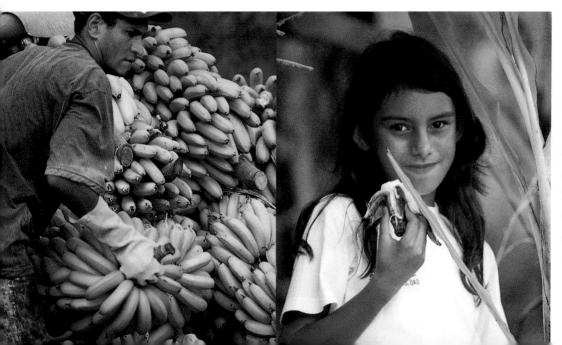

THE DIFFERENCES THAT COUNT

✤ Conventional plantations are often sprayed repeatedly with toxic pesticides and annual use can be over 15 times that of developed countries

✤ Up to 90 percent of aerially sprayed pesticides are lost to the atmosphere. Severe environmental damage to fish and coral results from the intensive use of artificial pesticides

✤ Blue plastic bags impregnated with pesticides usually cover bunches of conventional bananas. The bags are left scattered around and often end up in waterways. Systemic pesticides may be used that cannot be washed off the banana's skin and may linger in the fruit

✤ Conventional banana cultivation has resulted in one of the highest rates of deforestation in the world

✤ Workers on conventional plantations do not always have adequate protective clothing or know how to use pesticides safely, and children working on the plantations are exposed to them daily.

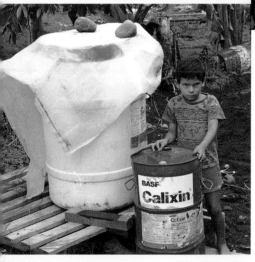

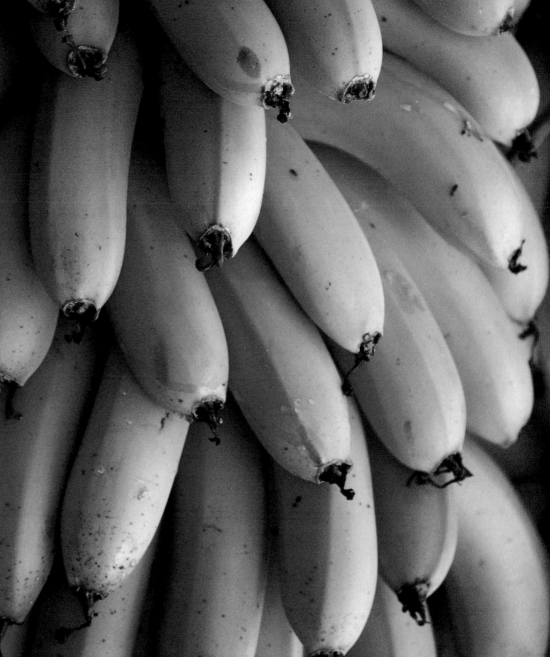

nitrogen-fixing trees are planted to help build soil fertility and provide shade. Weeding is done by hand with machetes. Ribbons are tied on to the new organic fruits so that they can be picked at the same stage of maturity. They are picked green but are not sprayed with the post-harvest chemicals that are used to delay ripening in conventional banana production.

Bunches are cut and graded, then loaded into refrigerated containers ready to begin their journey to the consumer. At biodynamic banana plantations such as the Finca Girasol plantation in the Dominican Republic, fruits and vegetables such as coconuts, corn, and sweet potatoes are integrated alongside goats, pigs, chickens, and bees to provide food for the workers.

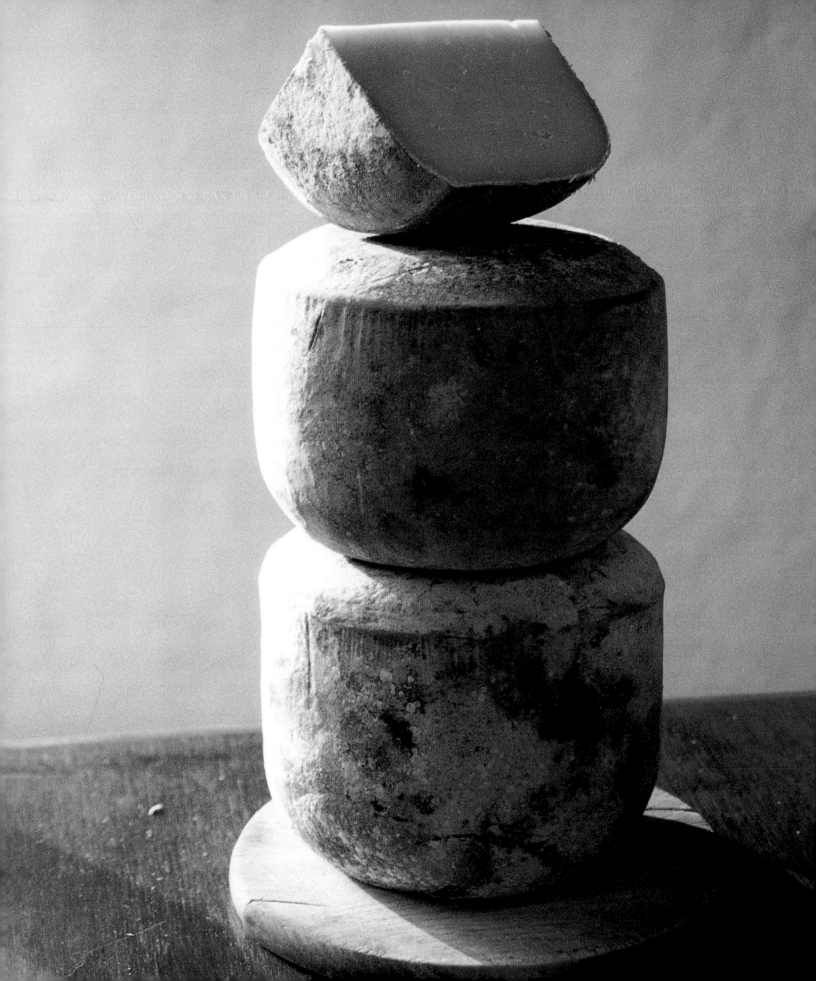

Making a meal of it

When it comes to putting food on their plates, thousands of consumers are discovering that organic foods offer the tastiest, healthiest, and best way forward, with the added reassurance of farm-to-plate traceability.

Our health and vitality depend on eating as wide a variety as possible of natural foods and wholesome staples, such as fruit and vegetables and good bread. Despite improvements to the way our food is being produced, only organic farming offers a complete package of "feel-good" benefits.

MAKING THE CHANGE TO ORGANIC

Changing to an organic diet does not need to happen overnight. Rather, experiment and try whatever you feel like. Organic breads of every description are now part of everyday life. So, too, are organic dairy products. With a growing number of dairy farmers going organic, there is ever-increasing availability and choice for everyone. Already in the US the daily organic quart of milk can be found on many supermarket shelves. Organic yogurts have been another success, representing a six percent share of the total British yogurt market. A British brand, Yeo Valley, is now market leader for natural yogurt, outselling all conventional brands there. And there are organic cheeses from mild goat's cheeses and nutty cheddars to the finest Parmesan.

A BETTER TASTE AND PEACE OF MIND

After decades of food scares culminating in bovine spongiform encephalopathy (BSE), coupled with worries over genetically modified organisms (GMOs) in animal feeds and animal welfare issues, organic meat offers consumers both peace of mind and high-quality, fuller-flavored meat. Many small producers are well established, and the challenge is now being met to develop systems that will enable organic meat to be produced on a larger scale.

Fish is a special case. Industrialized fishing methods and pollution have led to severe depletion of our fishing stocks and contaminated our fish. Intensive fish-farming has reduced the once noble salmon and trout to the status of the factory-farmed chicken. Organic farmed fish standards are being developed to help reverse this situation.

ORGANIC STANDARDS

There are strict regulations, enshrined in law, governing all aspects of organic food production (see page 244):

❖ All producers of organic foods must be certified by a recognized certification body and undergo a rigorous annual inspection by qualified inspectors

❖ Standards cover every aspect of food production, such as growing, packaging, processing, and transportation

❖ Full audited records of every stage ensure complete traceability from farm to table

❖ Each certification body has an official certification number or logo that appears on the packaging and is the consumer's guarantee of authenticity

From field to plate

From the milk in your tea or coffee to the jam on your toast, your scrambled eggs and bacon, or healthy muesli – the organic option is yours.

Organic breads that have real flavor and depth, and that you can sink your teeth into, are one of life's basic necessities. For variety, choose a different kind every week. Do the same with the excellent range of organic cereals and immediately breakfast becomes more interesting: rich, nutty, and competely natural, with no unwanted artificial extras. Kids love organic cornflakes and crunchies, while grown-ups with busy days ahead of them might prefer organic oatmeal.

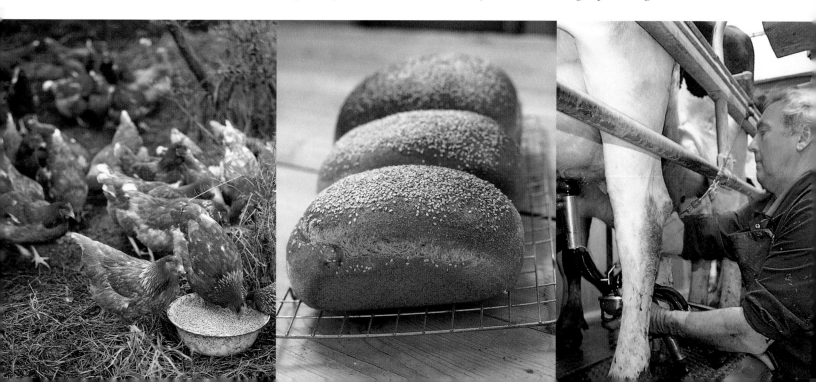

TOP BREAKFAST TIPS

✤ Organic soy milk, rice milk, and almond milk drinks are creamy, dairy-free alternatives for the milk jug

✤ Organic toast is given an extra lift spread with organic jams or marmalades – many are sweetened with honey, apple juice, or agave syrup instead of sugar

✤ Organic yogurts make light work of light breakfasts – they are deeply creamy and come in every flavor under the sun

✤ Chopped organic fruit, organic honey, and thick organic Greek yogurt make a breakfast made in heaven

An organic breakfast offers you the best possible start to the day and gives you that feel-good lift that comes from food you know you can trust.

Wake up to organics

Bread and milk are among life's basics, and for many people they offer the perfect start to the day. Organic bread and milk are prime examples of how organic farming can produce better quality daily staples.

Organically baked bread is the natural alternative for people who care about their health and the environment. Made from flour milled exclusively from organically grown grains, it contains none of the various dough improvers and additives that have become the hallmark of many mass-produced breads.

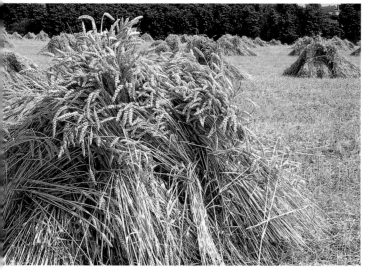

better bread

There is now available every conceivable variety of organically produced bread and baked goods you could possibly want to try, from everyday breads to handcrafted loaves, including gluten-free varieties. Everybody's taste and idea of the perfect loaf varies. The standard supermarket organic loaf is made to be more like a conventional loaf, and may contain organic soy flour, fat or sugar, or added vitamin C. The choice is yours – and will be reflected in the price you pay. Organic breads, made with extraordinary dedication by artisan bakers, include those from the Village Bakery in Cumbria, England, for example,

which has collected numerous awards for its excellent breads and cakes. As well as producing organic breads, the Village Bakery has an award-winning restaurant, a mail-order catalogue, runs bread-making courses, and is opening its own organic education center for the public. Its founder, Andrew Whitley, is typical of organic bakers in his belief that bread is the true staff of life and that the best bread requires nothing more than excellent organic flour, natural leavens – "mothers" – or yeast, salt, and time. Village Bakery breads are thus made with traditional long fermentations, avoiding the added enzymes which, although not declared on the label, are present in mass-produced bread. Baking the loaves in a wood-fired oven gives them a fine, moist texture, and the long fermentation

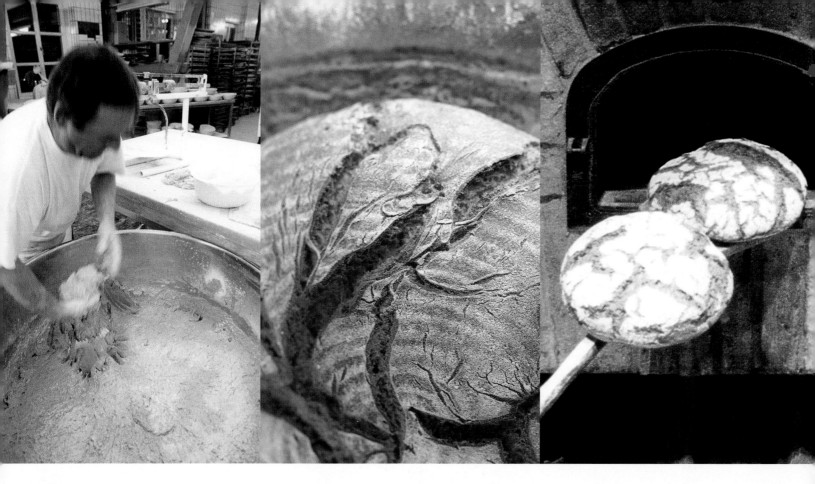

the producers

THE MASTER BAKERS

All bakeries producing organic bread and baked goods must be certified by an approved certification body such as The Independent Organic Inspectors Association and keep detailed records providing a full audit trail of all ingredients bought. In addition to the bakery premises being certified, the recipe for every single loaf or baked item must also be submitted, approved, and certified. Many of the small organic bread producers, such as the Authentic Bread Company, the Sunshine Organic bakery, Paul's, the Brilliant Bread Company, the Celtic Baker, and the Engine Shed, all in Great Britian, make bread in the time-honored way, using no more than a few simple, organic ingredients.

THE DIFFERENCES THAT COUNT

❖ All organic baked goods contain 95 percent or more organic ingredients
❖ Only a few natural baking aids, such as vitamin C, calcium carbonate, and rising agents, are permitted
❖ No hydrogenated fats, refined white sugars, artificial additives, or dough improvers may be used
❖ No GM ingredients are used

A field of organic wheat and a loaf of bread made with patience and integrity bring long-lasting joy and satisfaction.

ANDREW WHITLEY, MANAGING DIRECTOR, THE VILLAGE BAKERY

Wake up to organics

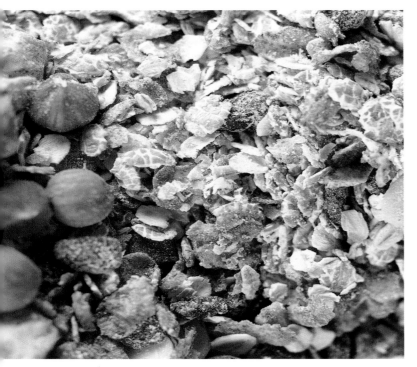

Nature's lesson

"The wholesomeness of the food we eat takes its root from the purity and freshness of its ingredients, leaving your body and mind in complete harmony. By placing science as an almighty, powerful means of control of nature, it is not only foolish but extremely dangerous. It is disappointing to see that man has not yet learned from his mistakes."

RAYMOND BLANC,
CHEF/PATRON,
LE MANOIR AUX QUAT' SAISONS

chickens, and outdoor pigs, and grow a range of organic vegetables for their local boxed food plans. In contrast to conventional cereals which are grown on an industrial scale, the cereals in Pertwood Farm mueslis are grown in rotation, deriving nourishment from composted manures and clover-rich pastures. Chickens and pigs are built into the rotation, providing extra soil fertility and helping to keep the weeds down. Pertwood's Mark Houghton Brown sums up the typical organic approach to farming: "Organic farming is not about returning to 'what farmers used to do', but about understanding how to continue to grow better crops and animals without using pesticides or artificial fertilizers. An organic farm is a specially managed part of the natural environment. We try to work with nature instead of fighting against it and understand that people are an intimate part of the biosphere, not isolated."

daily milk

The starting point for all organic dairy products is organic milk. This comes from organically raised cows that graze organic pastures supplemented with natural feeds and that receive no routine

adds to their complexity. Where a loaf of industrially baked bread from start to finish can take less than an hour and a half to make, theirs, and others like them, take anything from four to twenty-four hours – as you can tell by the flavor and deeply satisfying texture.

muesli

Organic mueslis are full of the grains of goodness that have nourished us from our beginnings. They are available loose or prepackaged, and there are many varieties and organic brands to try, such as Whole Earth Swiss Muesli, Nature's Path, Suma, Essential, Infinity Foods, Community, and Evernat. At Pertwood Farm, in the UK, they go one better. Their mueslis, which are wheat-, dairy-, and sugar-free, are made from their own organic oats, rye, and barley. Like organic farms everywhere, Pertwood offers plenty for consumers to feel good about. They preserve 330 acres of ancient pasture, raise pedigree Welsh Black and Hereford cattle, and rare Wiltshire Horns sheep, have laying

antibiotics. In the UK an organic dairy cow produces, on average, around 1,100 to 1,300 gallons (5,000 to 6,000 litres) of milk a year. Herd sizes vary from tiny herds to large dairy farms. None are pushed to produce milk to the limit of their genetic potential and day-to day management of the herds is designed to optimize the health of each cow. The result is clean, sweet-tasting milk that is delicious to drink, and from which a full range of organic dairy products is made.

cooperatives

Many organic dairy farmers and manufacturers, including Duchy Home Farm (*see page 40*) and Yeo Valley, are members or supporters of the Organic Milk Suppliers Cooperative (OMSCo). Run by farmers for farmers, OMSCo is the UK's leading organic milk marketing organization. Like similar organizations, it has helped to develop the organic market through its fairly traded policies and vision. OMSCo collects and markets the milk, gives technical advice to organic farmers, and those in conversion, and acts as the guardian of organic dairy-farming standards. All their farmers receive the same guaranteed price for their milk, helping their businesses to develop and grow. The OMSCo motto, "putting the heart back into farming", sums up what all organic farmers believe in. Their logo appears on many product brands.

local matters

Members cooperate in other ways too. To encourage the development and growth of local brands and outlets for milk and to help minimize transportation costs and food miles, OMSCo has recently formed Scottish and Welsh branches that enable local supporters to decide where their milk is to be sold and processed.

Manor Farm in Dorset, England, which has been farming organically since 1986 and whose organic milk is on sale in supermarkets, combines milk from other local OMSCo members with its own, ensuring its brand's true regional provenance. Manor Farm has also recently joined forces with a neighboring organic farm trust, the A. H. Warren Trust, which is now packing the milk for the farm. In addition, Manor Farm grows a traditional variety of wheat – Maris Widgeon – that provides straw for local thatchers. The wheat itself is sold to the local mill, Cann Mills, which grinds it to supply local bakers with locally grown organic flour.

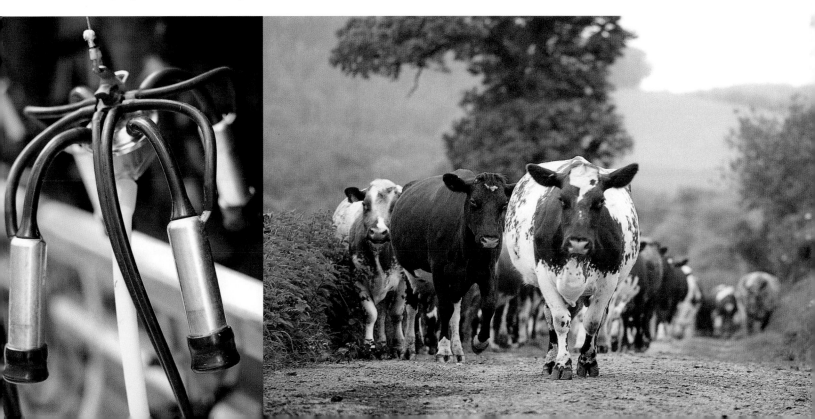

LUNCH

From field to plate

You don't need a long shopping list to create a delicious organic lunch: just a couple of fresh, light ingredients supplemented with those from the pantry.

Organic salads provide the perfect organic seasonal lunch. Topping them with a slice of organic goat's cheese, grilled until melted, turns any salad into an instant feast. Adding superfoods such as avocado, bean sprouts, pumpkin, or sunflower seeds, broccoli, or grated carrot will keep your vitamin levels high. Organic bulgur and couscous have full, nutty flavors and make easy, delicious pilafs and salads. For extra flavor, stir in a little spice paste and add a few organic raisins or some slivers of dried organic apricots. Organic pita bread stuffed with any kind of salad mix or homemade organic salsa are winners with everyone at any time of the year.

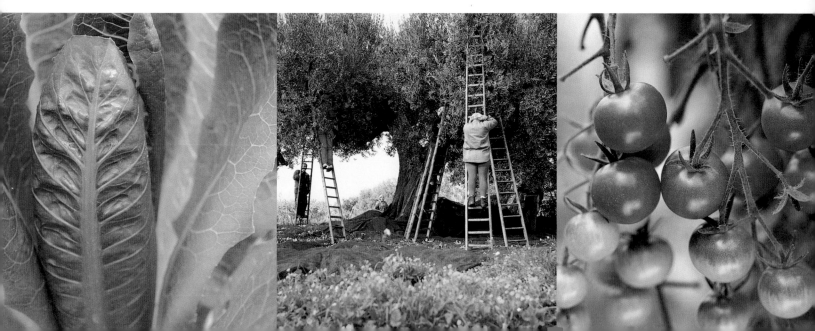

TOP LUNCH TIPS

✤ Natural nutritious winter warmers include organic baked potatoes, a chunk of roasted organic winter squash, or a simple dish of creamy polenta served with crumbled organic blue cheese

✤ If you do not feel like making your own lunch, browse organic deli counters and refrigerated and frozen food aisles for organic soups, salads, sandwiches, tofu burgers, vegetable tarts, and pizzas

✤ Organic liquid lunches provide a nutritious stopgap when time is short. The healthiest lunch of all is one you have juiced yourself: nature's health and vitality in a glass. Bottled organic juices are also excellent "pick-me-ups" (*see page 106*)

For formal lunches, fresh organic fish is the ultimate treat. Team it with an organic salad, sprigs of organic watercress, and a few organic new potatoes and your lunch is complete.

Let's do lunch

It has never been easier to enjoy a light, delicious, and healthy organic lunch that will nourish and sustain you throughout the day. Cheese and fish are tasty and nutritious, and now you can choose organic too.

Organic cheeses are made from organic milk and flavored, when required, with organic ingredients. Organic dairies may be anything from small, family-run concerns or cooperatives to large dairies producing well-known organic dairy brands for both the home and export markets. In the US, as elsewhere, there are shining examples of both large- and small-scale producers, and visiting a small organic cheese maker on vacation, for instance, is an education and inspiration in itself. It gives you an opportunity to try organic cheeses at their best, and to see at first hand the difference that the organic farming ethos can make.

small is great

One of the inspirational British small organic dairies is Loch Arthur in the county of Dumfries and Galloway, Scotland. Loch Arthur is a Camphill Community, which means that it is a member of an international movement of community villages that farm biodynamically, where people with special needs live and work alongside co-workers and every member of the community is valued equally. Altogether there are 90 communities throughout 20 countries, with 47 in Britain and Ireland. At Loch Arthur, good food is a way of life and everything is produced with love and care and respect for the environment. Produced from native Ayrshire cows, Loch Arthur's cheeses have won national acclaim. Like many organic craft cheesemakers, such as Llangloffan Farm in Wales, Old Plaw Hatch Farm in West Sussex, and Duddlewell Dairy in East Sussex, the Loch Arthur dairy favors unpasteurized milk because of its health-giving benefits and the extra nuances of flavor it has. The farm also produces hand-churned butter, yogurts, muesli, and honey, runs a boxed organic meat program and has its own organic bakery and shop.

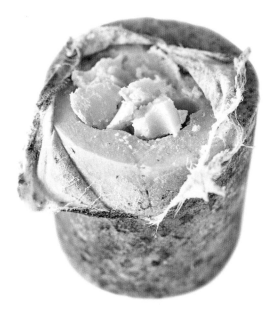

big is beautiful

Organic dairies can also be big and beautiful, too. Two that are in the UK, Rachel's Dairy in Wales and Yeo Valley in Somerset, prove that it is possible to remain true to your principles, produce food with integrity and be successful in big business too. Both producers have dedicated organic dairies and are fully committed to developing the organic market in the long term. Graham Keating of Yeo Valley is justifiably proud of their achievements: "Conventional modern trading relationships and the demands of City institutions are damaging significant sections of the rural economy. The conventional dairy industry is but one casualty of a trading system that destroys rather than nurtures its suppliers. We believe in the organic way and the kind of ground-breaking initiatives we have developed with the Organic Milk Suppliers Co-operative (*see page 77*) provide an opportunity to redress this awful mess. Cooperation and mutual support is the way forward and enables ever greater numbers of consumers to enjoy our organic products."

fish dishes

The development of organic farmed fish (*see right*) is in its infancy and has resulted from consumer demand for better-quality fish and better deal for the fish we eat. Standards have been

the producers

Thanks to two pioneering trout farmers in Great Britian, Nigel Woodhouse in Hawkshead, Cumbria, and his friend Tim Small in Lechlade, Gloucestershire, the tale of organic trout is a happy one. Switching to organic changed these men's lives, making them feel happier and proud again to be fish farmers. Local sales are booming and both are supplying supermarkets. The key to organic farmed fish is freedom of space, which alleviates the need to suppress disease, and which means their fishes' own immune systems can function well. For Tim Small this has meant cutting his stock densities to one fifth of their earlier levels, with dramatic effects. Previously his trout were dull in color and apathetic by nature. Because they were crammed so close, they were more susceptible to infections. Now his fish, like Nigel's, are alert, healthy, have a handsome blue sheen, and are well spotted. Their fish have a real flavor and are naturally pink, due to feeding on the wild shrimp found in the streams that flow through their trout ponds. Whereas these producers used to kill 5,000 trout at a time, which were then left to asphyxiate, the trout are now stunned humanely, a few at a time, and are fresher. As Tim Small explains, "Twenty-five years ago, trout-farming was a cottage industry, now it's a cut-throat business. Wholesalers are only interested in paying the lowest price and once you get locked into the intensive spiral, the only way you can survive is to find ways of squeezing more fish out of the system. Farming organically has reversed that. I'm happy, so are my trout, and so are my customers."

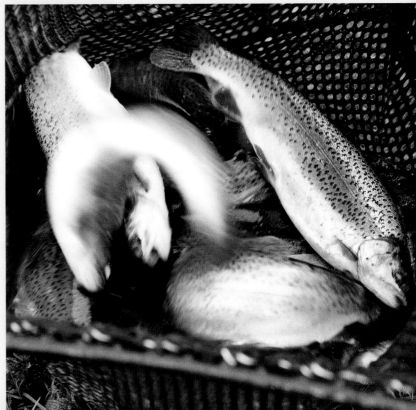

Let's do lunch

developed by the Soil Association in the UK and Naturland in Germany. The aims were to produce the best possible conditions for the fish, minimize adverse effects on the environment and provide the highest-quality fish for the consumer. Fish scientists, environmentalists, fishermen, and Compassion In World Farming were all consulted and standards were established covering every aspect of fish breeding, rearing, and management, water quality, environmental impact, and the encouragement of local resources.

Salmon and trout are two of the world's most popular fish. In the Orkneys and in Ireland organically farmed salmon have far more space than regular farmed fish. They live in waters that are carefully monitored for purity and have powerful natural tides to swim against. Organic salmon feed contains far less oil than conventional feed, allowing the fish to put on weight naturally and slowly. Adding crushed shrimp shells rather than artificial colorings to their feed gives them their salmon-pink hue. No pesticides or routine medication are used, and the fish are individually culled by hand, which is swift and less stressful.

The eating quality of organically farmed fish is quite striking and many people find that the fish have more flavor and

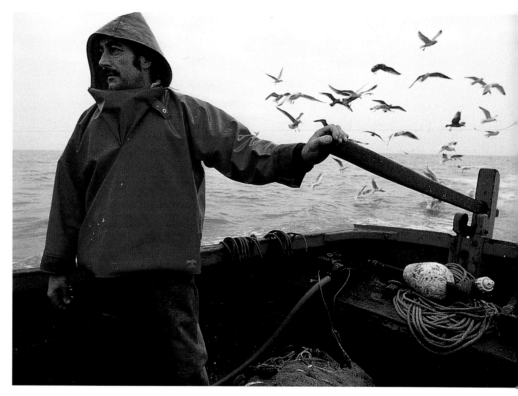

better texture and are less flabby and oily. In every way they represent a return to how farmed fish should be.

THE DIFFERENCES THAT COUNT

✤ Organically farmed fish live in exceptionally pure waters and are stocked in extremely low densities, so that they occupy no more than 1.5 percent of the water available
✤ Organically farmed salmon have strong water currents to swim against
✤ Organically farmed fish are given only high-quality natural organic feed
✤ There is no use in organic fish-farming of pesticides, routine antibiotics, or any kind of artificial coloring

fish for life

Most sea fish are caught in large quantities in modern fishing boats that can remain at sea for several days. Local fishermen who sell that day's catch are becoming a rarity. Buying local fish when you can and supporting fish-sellers

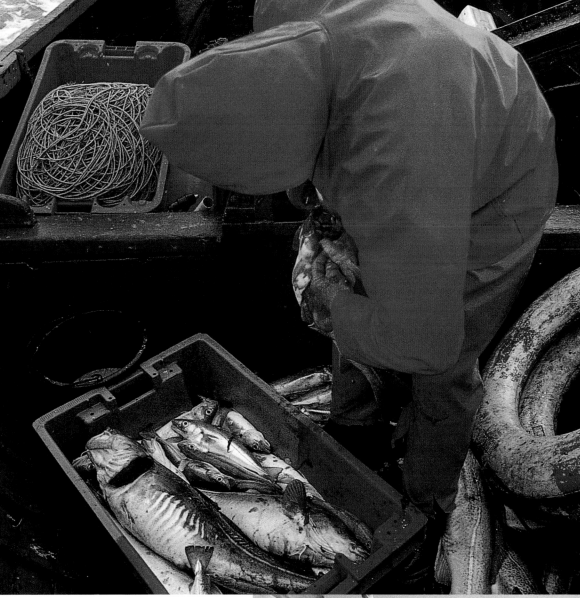

The real cost

"The real cost of food is not the price we pay in the shops. We have recently calculated that the external costs caused by modern agriculture amount to over £2.3 billion every year. This includes £120 million from contamination of drinking water with pesticides, £106 million from soil erosion and organic carbon losses, and £125 million from damage to wildlife and habitats: a hidden subsidy of £208 for each hectare [two acres] of arable and permanent pasture in the UK. For every kilogram [2 lbs] of pesticide used in farming, it costs £8.60 to clean up the costs. Those farmers that do not pollute or do things that negatively affect human health or the environment, do not receive this hidden subsidy. It is a perverse situation, as the polluters win."

PROFESSOR JULES PRETTY,
DIRECTOR, CENTRE FOR
ENVIRONMENT AND SOCIETY,
UNIVERSITY OF ESSEX

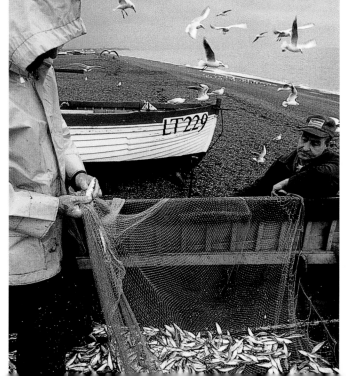

who buy their fish from day trawlers are two ways to help support sustainable fishing. In the UK fishing community of St. Helena in the South Atlantic, fish from the pure waters around the island are caught using rods and lines. They are then processed on the island, so the economic benefit goes directly to the community. Fish For Life is a similar operation here in North America involving the traditional fisherfolk of Alaska. You can also buy fish locally in small fishing communities.

DINNER

From field to plate

Dinner is the main meal of the day for many people and whether it is a simple supper, a family meal, or a celebration, organic food makes it special.

Organic production methods and foods speak for themselves and have true integrity. All there is left for you to do is enjoy them and rejoice in the fact that the organic dinner option is now a reality for everyone. As for ingredients, the world is your organic oyster – you will always be able to find something to suit your taste and mood. You might choose to make a creamy risotto with organic leeks and red peppers, go oriental and stir-fry, make your own organic pizza, produce a homey hot pot, or settle for organic sausage and eggs or a ready-made vegetarian korma. A simple roast chicken is sublime and will yield plenty of tasty pickings and superb organic stock.

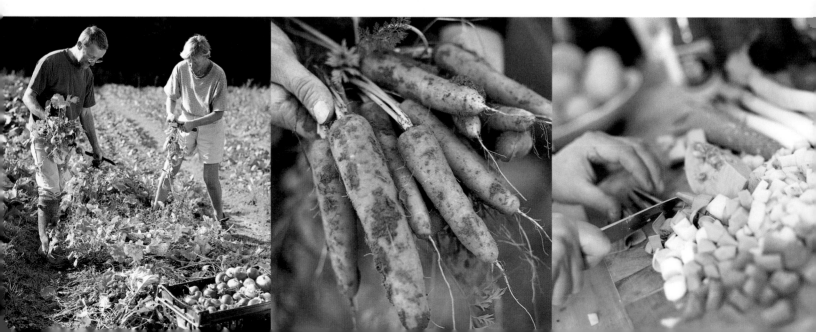

TOP DINNER TIPS

✤ Chunky-cut organic vegetables, tossed in organic olive oil then roasted in the oven, are full of flavor and are great with meat, fish, and grain dishes

✤ Mini organic roasts are perfect for two and are quick and easy to do

✤ Organic beef or pork stroganov – strips of meat cooked briefly with fried organic mushrooms and finely chopped shallots, mustard, and crème fraîche – is an instant, delicious way to make your organic prime cuts go further

✤ For comfort suppers, organic risottos are the new pasta: include whatever vegetables are in season

Cooking is far more enjoyable when your food has true taste and integrity. Organic foods add that extra dimension and mean your dinner will be truly appetizing.

Prime time

Whether you want a sizzling roast or a simple stir-fry, choosing organic ingredients will help to ensure that your meal is one to remember and that it has been produced in a wholesome, natural way.

Organic farmers are passionate about producing real food and about animal welfare (*see pages 28 and 37*). For many established organic producers, this is

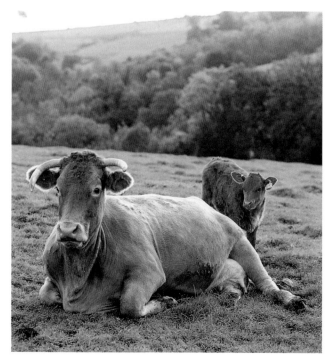

reflected in the quality and taste of their meat and represents in many ways a return to how meat should be. Animal welfare comes at a price. This makes organic meat dearer than conventional meat, although this can often be offset by buying cheaper cuts, making expensive cuts go further by adding other organic ingredients and buying from local organic farmers. Whether you sizzle or simmer, organic meat is precious. Fresh meat should look dry and smell sweet. For flavor, buy properly hung meat with the correct proportion of fat. If buying meat by mail

order, do not be afraid to ask as many questions as you like, and if buying frozen meat, choose vacuum-sealed packs.

prime quality

Since organic meat grows at a natural, unforced rate, it often has more flavor and a firmer texture than you may be used to, making it more satisfying to eat. Because traditional breeds are used more, pork, for example, may have extra back fat, while beef can have extra marbling. This is a sign of quality. The fat provides valuable flavor and added succulence, and can be cut off before eating. Flavor also depends on hanging times. Chicken, for example, is definitely improved by hanging for a few days in the traditional way. Organic meat from supermarkets is often aged less and will be more uniform in texture and taste than that from a local producer or butcher. As with nonorganic meat, the tender premium cuts command a premium price, while braising cuts such as shoulder offer much better value. Organic sausages and burgers are popular and generally offer good value. If you do not feel like cooking, there are many prepared organic meals available.

state-of-the-art caring

Organic farmers care deeply about animal welfare. Many established organic producers around the world, and from all over the country, share this passion which is reflected in the taste and quality of their meat. Organic farming is also about finding new solutions and wherever it is practiced you will find ground-breaking initiatives that are moving organic farming forward to even greener pastures. Chicken and pork are a case in point: since we have become used to low prices for chicken and pork, the development of these meats organically – where the differences in the cost of raising them and in animal welfare is most acute – has been slow. Two organic farms in England, Eastbrook Farm (*see right*) and Sheepdrove Farm, have started to change this. Sheepdrove Farm produces 1,000 chickens a week. From the minute they arrive as day-old chicks, they

Working together

"Our goal and vision as organic farmers is to build a lasting relationship with the soil and land we farm, and the people we produce for. As farmers, our responsibility is to produce the best food possible for consumers, in a way that cares for the countryside and farm animals. As consumers, we can help by supporting the farmers who take these responsibilities seriously. Then together we will be able to create a sustainable future for ourselves and our planet."

HELEN BROWNING OBE,
CHAIRMAN, THE SOIL ASSOCIATION
AND FARMER, EASTBROOK FARM

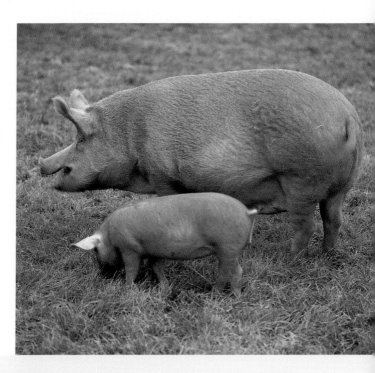

the producers

PREMIUM PORK

A role model for all that organic farming can achieve, Eastbrook Farm is one of the best-known organic farms in the UK. Their organic meat, sausages, and traditionally cured bacon can be found on many supermarket shelves. Over the last ten years they have developed a pork production system that is second to none and has become a blueprint for the emerging organic pork industry.

Visit the farm and you will see alert, contented pigs glowing with health. They live in small groups, have clean, mobile houses and, unlike most outdoor pigs, are moved around constantly onto

fresh pastures. Piglets stay with their mothers as long as possible and the very highest standards of animal husbandry ensure that any illness is kept to a minimum. Antibiotics are used only in emergencies. Pigs are slaughtered as close as possible to the farm. Eastbrook Farm has an ongoing research program to find ways to improve every aspect of production and eating quality. Recently, they joined forces with one of the UK's leading free-range pork producers and processors, offering long-term contracts to encourage more pig farmers to convert and to fast-forward the development of organic pork.

Prime time

receive five-star treatment. They are housed in modern, mobile French chicken houses and range, completely free, as far as the eye can see on fresh, green pasture, supplemented with organic feed that contains home-grown grain. The pasture contains a rich mix of clover, sheep's parsley, yarrow, chicory, salad burnet, and bird's foot trefoil, from which the chickens derive essential minerals. The quality shows in their sunshine-tinged skins. They live twice as long as conventional raised chickens – until 12 weeks old – and are killed and processed on the farm with minimum stress. The results are great: chickens with real flavor, moist breasts, and meaty legs.

oodles of noodles

Walk into any organic store, anywhere in the world, and you will find a wide range of organic noodles. These include classic Italian pastas and pastas made from ancient varieties of kamut and spelt wheat. There are also Asian rice noodles, silky-smooth Japanese buckwheat noodles, and "new-age" types made with different grains such as corn, millet, or soy, developed for the growing market of people allergic to wheat. As intensive farming methods dominate the production of the world's staple grains, especially wheat, organic pastas, and noodles, like bread, have a particularly important role to play. Buying them helps support and develop sustainable grain-growing methods and means that you get pasta or noodles produced more naturally. They come in all shapes, sizes, and flavors and can be bought fresh or dried at prices to fit all budgets. Some are made by artisan craftsmen in traditional ways and some are made

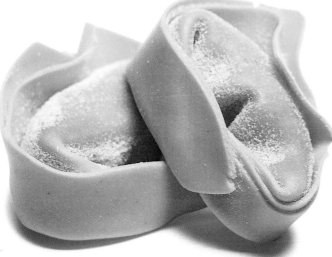

in modern factories for the mass market, but all are made exclusively from organic grains.

pasta craft

Our love of Italian pasta and pasta dishes means that organic pastas dominate the shelves in many supermarkets and health food stores. The finest pastas are made using traditional methods in which the pasta is made using bronze cutters and dried slowly at low temperatures. Many small Italian organic pasta manufacturers, such as the Campo and La Terra e Il Cielo cooperatives, and the Barbagallo family in Fiumefreddo, Sicily, use this technique. The Barbagallo family grow their own organic durum wheat and, to preserve maximum flavor and vitality, grind it when fresh and mix it with pure mountain water in their own mill. The Sakuri family, who live in the foothills of the Japanese Alps, use the same method, but air-dry their organic noodles over bamboo rods for 30 hours. Major organic brands specializing in organic pasta and pasta sauces, such as Seeds of Change, can also take great care. Their organic spaghetti, penne, and gemelli pastas are made in Italy from locally-grown organic durum wheat, using the same traditional methods.

LIQUID GOLD

Organic olive oil is indispensable to a modern diet and a joy to use. Unlike conventional olive oils, whether everyday or premium estate-bottled, all are cold-pressed, and almost all are extra-virgin oil, which is the highest grade of olive oil. Like good wine, each oil has its own character depending on the variety of olives used to make the oil and where it is grown – from the delicate, mellow, sweet, green, or golden oils of Spain and France to the robust Greek oils and the intense, green, fruity oils of Tuscany. Have an everyday olive oil on hand for your cooking and a premium oil to make salad dressings and aïoli (garlic mayonnaise), to drizzle over cooked vegetables, and to mash into potatoes. In this way you can discover the diverse world of organic olive oils for yourself. Other organic oils to try include safflower, sunflower, and sesame, and delicious organic nut oils such as walnut or hazelnut. Again, all are cold-pressed to preserve maximum nutritional value and have the full flavor of the seed or nut from which they were pressed. Because of this you need very little. Hermetically sealed organic designer oils, brimming with essential omega fatty acids, are highly recommended by various health "gurus" and specialists as they ensure you get the right amount of these all-important fatty acids. They must be kept in the refrigerator and should never be heated.

THE DIFFERENCES THAT COUNT

✤ Organic olive producers (*see below*) tend to have smaller, traditional groves, where the olives are often picked by hand and crushed in their own or in local mills

✤ Organic olive groves are often situated at high altitudes, where pests are less of a problem and where the trees help to prevent soil erosion

✤ Growers of organic olives use biological controls such as hanging pheromone traps in the trees to monitor pests and grow nitrogen-fixing plants in between the trees to help provide soil fertility

✤ Organic regulations ensure pressing at the lowest temperatures to preserve maximum flavor and nutritional quality

the producers

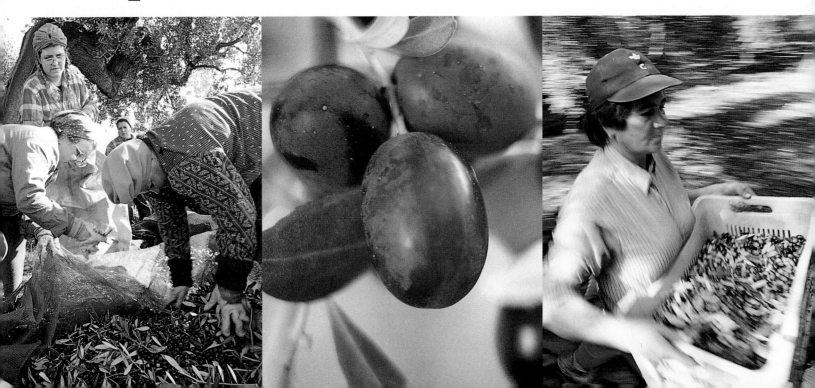

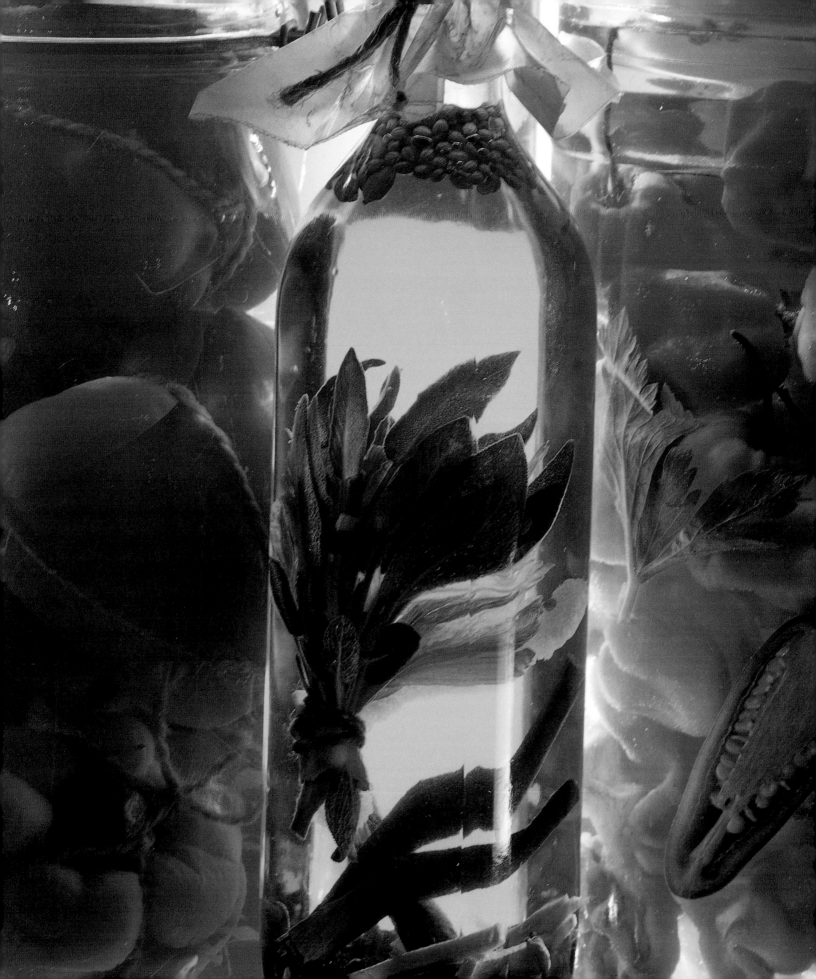

Your organic pantry

Whether you are rustling up an emergency meal in minutes or adding an essential ingredient to a recipe, the organic pantry contains those staple favorites on which you know you can rely.

The organic pantry is a special pantry. Not only will the contents of this pantry be made from certified organic foods and ingredients containing no artificial additives, but they will also have been processed in the best possible way, using just a few permitted processing aids (*see page 244*).

INSIDE THE ORGANIC PANTRY

All tastes are catered for and, if you want healthy alternatives, you will find them. You will also find all your everyday essentials, organic flavors from around the world, exotic treats and all your familiar favorites, including ketchup, mayonnaise, and baked beans. If you surf the internet you will find organic online shops listing even more options.

In all, over 3,000 different kinds of organic dried, processed, and convenience foods are already on the market for you to try. When you start to substitute just a few organic items, your pantry will become that bit more special.

MAKING THE CHANGE TO ORGANIC

Organic foods may be made by specialist organic manufacturers who only produce organic foods, or, by conventional manufacturers keen to offer an organic option. Whether they are dedicated organic producers or not, all of those manufacturing organic foods must be certified by an organic certification body such as Farm Verified Organic and inspected every year.

QUALITY COUNTS

Standards and regulations covering organic processed foods are very strict (*see right*). Organic ingredients must be verified and kept separate at all times, and if conventional lines are produced in the same factory, all equipment must be cleaned down before the organic products are made. As an extra precaution, organic lines are usually the first batch produced each day. In addition, any organic processed foods must adhere to all the usual food, safety and hygiene regulations.

ORGANIC STANDARDS

All processed foods labeled "organic" must be produced to the following standards and guidelines:

✤ All manufacturers of organic processed foods must be certified by an organic certification body

✤ All ingredients used in organic products must be kept separate from ingredients for use in conventional products at all times

✤ Detailed routine records, including cleaning and processing schedules, must be kept at all times and made available for audit by certification inspectors

✤ Any business that packs, processes or relabels organic products out of the sight of the customers must also be certified

A store
of treasures

The modern pantry is changing fast. These days it is designed
to be in tune with your lifestyle, and with so many organic options out
there you will find there is more than enough to suit you.

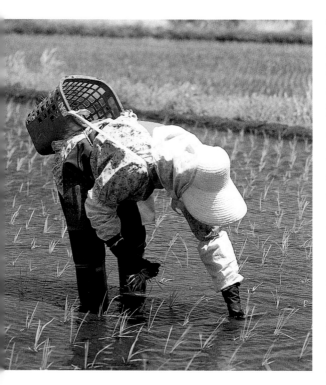

Whatever your lifestyle, your organic pantry is likely to have a few essential basics, be strong in Italian products and essential flavorings, and have a few lifesavers for emergencies. An organic comfort corner is a must, and if you have a sweet tooth, there is a wealth of organic options out there waiting for you to discover.

back to basics

Organic beans, legumes, grains, and dried pastas and noodles (*see page 88*) make cheap, simple, and nutritious meals. All your favorite types of rice are readily available, including wild, risotto, basmati, and fragrant Thai rice. Ready-cooked canned beans are ideal for when time is short, and precooked polenta and brown rice are popular standbys.

nuts & seeds

Organic nuts, seeds, and dried fruits offer an explosion of flavor. They are not coated with mineral oils or sulphur dioxide – one of the reasons why organic dried apricots are dark brown instead of bright orange. Organic sunflower, sesame, and pumpkin seeds are healthy snacks and ideal for scattering over salads or adding to grain dishes, and breads. Toasted sesame seeds are delicious: grind them for salad dressings, and use them in stir-fries and omelettes or over broccoli.

flour power

Most organic flours are milled by skilled craftsmen millers who are using traditional milling techniques. They produce unbleached, stone-ground flours, milled gently at low temperatures to retain the maximum possible nutritional content and flavor. Shipton Mill and Doves Farm, both in England, are Britain's two best-known organic millers producing organic flour that is widely available nationwide. Other millers that are producing organic flours on a smaller scale, include Little Salkeld Mill in Melmerby, Cumbria, Maud Foster Mill in Boston, Lincolnshire, and Thelnetham Windmill in Stanton, Suffolk.

al italia

Organic canned tomatoes, passatas, tomato purées, and olive oils (*see page 89*) are essential everyday ingredients. You can also buy bottled organic appetizers such as roast Italian vegetables under olive oil, *crema di aspergi* (creamed asparagus paté), artichoke hearts, capers, olives, balsamic vinegar, sun-dried tomatoes, and grissini. And if time is of the essence, why not try one of the many preprepared organic pasta sauces, adding your own touch with some chopped fresh basil or parsley.

wok organic

It is easy to add an organic eastern zest to your food. Organic Chinese sauces, teamed with chopped fresh ginger, garlic, scallions, and cilantro, make light work of wok cooking.

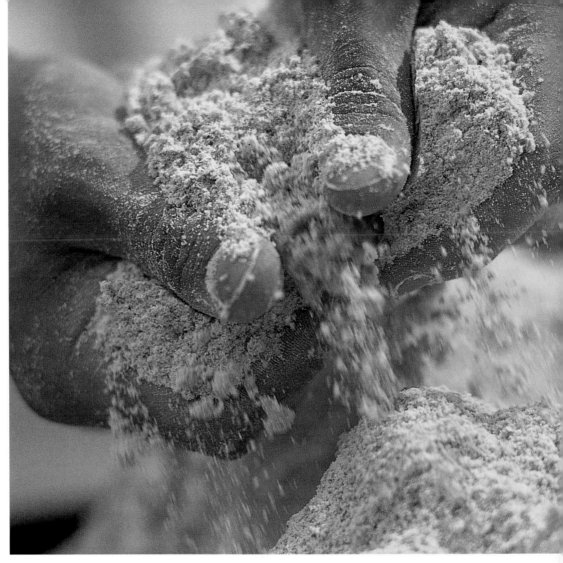

If spices are to your taste, there is an ever-increasing range of preprepared Indian spice pastes, sauces, and pickles to try. Japanese organic miso, shoyu, and tamari sauces are pure, natural, and authentic. These sauces can be used as a substitute for salt and contain beneficial enzymes that may help your digestive system.

salty tales

Every home should have a salt box. Natural sea salt, made in the age-old way from evaporated sea water, is nature's finest seasoning. It is soft and flaky and contains important trace elements, such as zinc, calcium, potassium, and iodine, that are normally removed from table salt during processing. Several, including the Anglesey sea salt, Halen Môn, which is already a favorite with top chefs, have been certified as organically pure. This guarantees that they have been produced from clean, uncontaminated sea water, that they contain none of the additives normally added to table salt to make it pour more easily and that they have undergone stringent monitoring for quality control.

A store of treasures

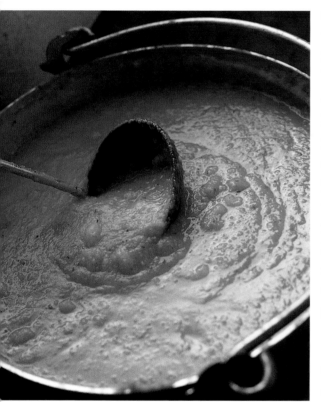

lifesavers

If you ever find yourself short of fresh food there are many organic emergency pantry options to consider.

Organic rice cakes come in a range of different flavors and are healthy, wheat-free, and snackable at all hours. Organic Mexican refried beans, canned hummus, canned beans, tacos, and salsas make instant lunches, dips, and salads. Soup (*see above*) is the ultimate lifesaver

and there are several organic brands to try, including Suma, Simply Organic, Seeds of Change, and Go Organic in the UK. Soup jars are recyclable and make excellent storage containers. If you feel like a quick snack or need an addition to your organic plowman's lunch, there are organic pickled onions, gherkins, piccalillis, and chutneys of all kinds. For vegans, Organic Valley's canned rice pudding is a dairy-free alternative, while Mrs. Moon's excellent range of muffin mixes – which also includes one for vegans – means you can have organic muffins for tea any time you want them.

getting saucy

The organic pantry offers many possibilities, including barbecue sauce, brown sauce, and organic tomato ketchup. For when you are feeling lazy there are also many excellent organic salad dressings, mayonnaises and good old-fashioned salad dressing as well.

sweet things

Those with a sweet tooth can take their pick from organic molasses, to dark-brown sticky sugars, demerara sugar, maple syrup, and honeys from around

the world (*see page 96*), or try alternative sweeteners such as barley, maize malt, and brown rice syrups. Organic jams, marmalades, and fruit spreads are made without refined white sugar, and some brands are sweetened with honey or apple juice – or go wild with organic lychee jam, blueberry spread, and vanilla jelly.

naughty but nice

Whether sweet or savory, there are occasions when only tried-and-tested comfort favorites will do. Try the organic alternatives and you may find them even more comforting. Start with stone-ground organic tortilla chips. They come in various flavors and are made from yellow and blue corn varieties. Both they and organic potato chips are fried in organic sunflower oil, as is organic popcorn. Chocoholics can take their pick of the many organic options on offer (*see right*), such as hot chocolate, chocolate cookies, and brownies. There is also a huge selection of organic cakes and cookies to choose from. Fruit, nut, and muesli bars can give you sustained energy, and organic lollipops and candies are fun and fruity.

meat-free too

The organic vegetarian and vegan are well catered for and new products that combine good nutrition with good taste are becoming available daily. They include several ranges of delicious patés and sandwich spreads, varied pestos, and a wide range of soy products, including tofu (*see page 100*).

superfoods

Pure organic "superfoods" for super health are gaining in popularity. These include hemp seed, spirulina, chlorella, wheatgrass, designer oils that give you the right balance of essential omega 3 and omega 6 fatty acids, and superfood supplement ranges such as Pure Synergy and The Missing Link. They are easy to add to your diet and pantry. Look out for them in health food shops and organic supermarkets and shops.

seaweeds

One of the up-and-coming super foods, seaweeds are among the richest sources of vitamins on earth. Organic seaweed comes from certified pure sources and is sustainably harvested. Use it for broths, salads, sushi, stir-fries, and with fish, or try organic seaweed table condiments, for sprinkling over all kinds of food. Seaweed food capsules are a natural organic nutritional supplement and a good foundation for health.

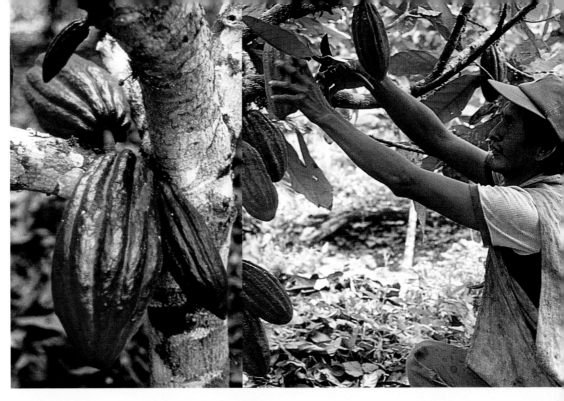

the producers

GUILT-FREE GOODIES

The organic option is one you need never feel guilty about, especially when it comes to chocolate. Most mass-produced chocolate contains refined white sugar, hydrogenated fats, and artificial flavorings. Organic chocolate does not, and it uses organic sugar and up to twice the amount of organic cocoa solids to give the chocolate its pure, rich taste. Organic cocoa is farmed sustainably. Like organic tea and coffee (*see page 104*), choosing organic leaves a better taste in your mouth altogether.

FAIR TRADE FEASTS

One of the leading organic chocolate brands, Green & Black's, was one of the first companies to popularize organic chocolate in the UK, and its Maya Gold chocolate was also the first product ever to carry the Fairtrade Mark (*see page 220*). Green & Black's trades directly with organic cocoa producers, offering them long-term contracts and paying a premium for their cocoa beans. Initiatives from pioneering companies such as this and from organizations such as Oxfam mean that choosing organic or fairly traded chocolate can make a real difference to the environment and to the lives of the people who grow the cocoa. The El Ceibo cooperative in Bolivia (*see above*) is an example of how, by selling their organic cocoa to Oxfam, some farmers are reaping additional benefits from Oxfam's fair trade initiatives and are guaranteed a fair deal.

Focus on honey

Made by bees receiving the best of care throughout their lives, organic honey is pure and natural and comes to you from around the world.

Organic honey comes from hives situated in remote and unpolluted areas, or those well away from any industrial sites or intensively managed farms and orchards, and undergoes no heating or other refining that can damage its nutritional content or flavor. No insecticides, antibiotics, or chemical repellents are used, the wood for the hives comes from untreated timbers, and organic beeswax is usually used to make the combs. Feeding the hives with sugar is forbidden, except in emergencies, and sufficient honey is left in the hives for the bees to feed on over winter.

a tale of two honeys

New Zealand has vast areas of unpolluted natural bushlands and landscapes, and is the world's leading high-quality organic honey producer. All sites are approved by the organic certifying body BIO-GRO, and beekeepers must produce Land User Statements guaranteeing that no toxic sprays are used in the area for a minimum distance of 3 miles (5 km). Every batch of honey is rigorously tested for residues to confirm purity. New Zealand's organic honey producers (*see below left*) are small, family concerns. Between 35–45 lb (15–20 kg) honey is left on each hive to feed the bees over winter and extraction is as natural as possible. The honey is never heated over natural hive temperature (100°F/38°C) nor is it finely filtered. This allows the precious pollen grains to be retained in the honey.

Organic "wild" honeys from tropical countries, such as Borneo, the Solomon Islands, Zambia, and India, are produced by traditional beekeepers, providing them with a valuable income and allowing them to continue with their traditional lifestyle. Many are also fairly traded (*see page 220*). Oxfam FairTrade honey from Zambia helps support the local economy. Trucks that come to collect the honey also deliver essentials such as salt and bicycle tires to the villages. As Mr. Bunonge, a producer in North Western province, Zambia, says: "We cannot survive on local sales alone. Exporting our honey to other countries and being able to sell through Oxfam is very important." Their traditional hives

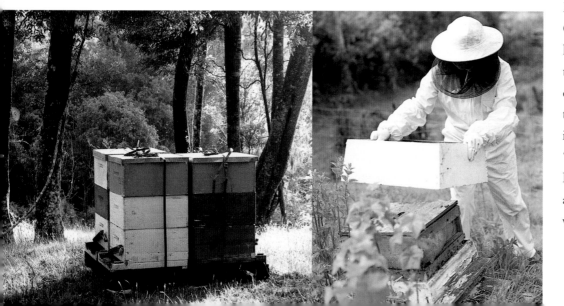

THE DIFFERENCES THAT COUNT

✤ Organic standards are very stringent, ensuring that organic honey is of the finest quality

✤ Organic honey comes from hives situated in remote and unpolluted areas. Each site has to be approved by an organic certification body

✤ No insecticides, antibiotics, or chemical repellents are used in the hives

✤ Organic honey undergoes no processing or refining that might damage both its nutritional content and flavor

✤ Hives are made from untreated wood and organic beeswax is usually used to make the combs

✤ The common practice of feeding the hives with sugar is generally forbidden and sufficient honey is left in the hives for the bees to feed on over winter

✤ Bees receive the best care throughout their lifecycles

✤ Organic honey is packed in recyclable glass jars

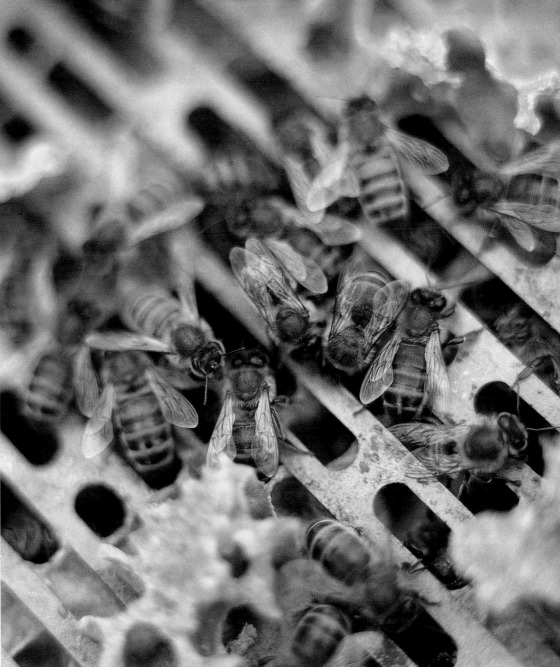

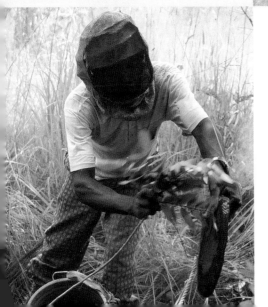

are made using forest materials. Bark is formed into cylinders and closed with a grass door. Hives are then hung in trees to protect bees from honey badgers and other predators. Harvesting is a perilous business. The beekeeper ties a bundle of leaves to a fiber rope and lights them to smolder to make the bees drowsy. He then extracts the honey by climbing the tree and scooping it out into a bucket, or breaking off sections of honeycomb to extract the honey once back on the ground (*see left*). Unlike commercially blended honeys, natural honeys, like wines, vary in taste and texture depending on the country and season in which they are produced, and the kind of flowers from which the bees collect the nectar.

Chill out

Freshly prepared chilled and frozen organic convenience foods are one of the fastest-growing sectors of the market. From pies to pizzas and soups to sorbets, ready-made has become an organic reality.

For regular organic eaters, this means not sacrificing your principles or taste buds when you do not feel like cooking, are in a hurry or need lunch ready to go.

organics to go

If you are new to organic food or have not sampled much yet, prepared meals are the ideal place to start. Generally, they are good value for money. The same stringent organic regulations apply, including full organic traceability of all raw materials, and washing down work surfaces with drinkable water every day, so you can be sure your take-out meal is as organic and pure as possible. Organic take-out foods will all have the certification logo on the packaging. Also, many shops, one-stop retail chains and cafés are now producing take-out foods that are made with organic ingredients, although they will not be sold as organic if they and the premises are not certified.

deli delights

At the delicatessen counters you will find organic salamis and hams, patés, sun-dried tomatoes, quiches, various pies, and often organic cakes sold by the slice.

ready-made

Head for refrigerated and frozen food aisles in organic supermarkets or major retail supermarkets and, depending on the store, you will find all sorts, including seasonal organic soups and stocks, fresh pasta and pasta sauces, smoked fish, tofu products, prepared salads, pizzas, children's meals, desserts, and even organic custard. There are organic prepared main meals to give you a taste of different cuisines from around the world, from macaroni and cheese to vegetable tagine with couscous, and from vegetable chow mein to chicken dhansak. Prepared meals are suitable for conventional ovens or microwaves, and vegetarians are very well catered to.

freezer fare

The range of frozen organic foods grows daily, including homey fare such as shepherd's pie and vegetarian lasagnes, pizzas, frozen vegetables, organic ice creams (*see right*), sorbets, and frozen desserts. In a bid to make organic food more affordable, the food retailer Iceland has converted its entire range of own-label frozen vegetables and tub ice

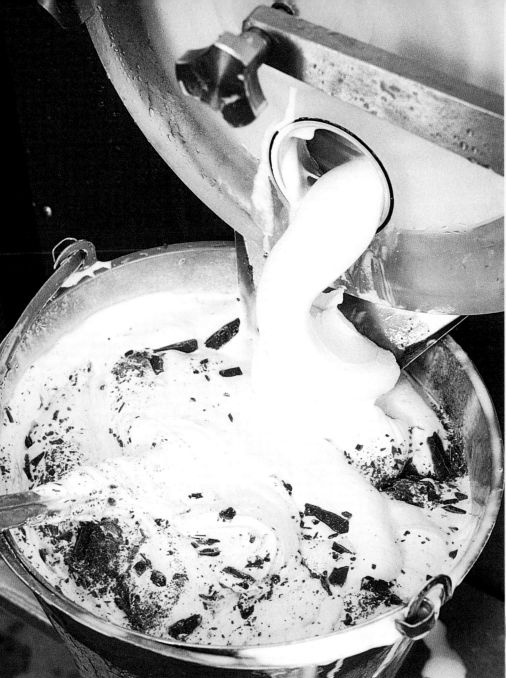

COLD COMFORT

Like organic chocolate, organic ice cream is one treat you can indulge in without feeling too guilty. This is especially the case when it is made by producers such as the original organic ice cream dairy, Rocombe Farm Ice cream in England (*see left and below*), or other small British producers such as the September Dairy in Herefordshire, Cream O' Galloway in Dumfries and Galloway, Scotland, or Green & Black's in London. All these ice creams are made in the traditional way from cream, eggs, milk, real fruit, real flavorings, and sugar. If stabilizers are required, only natural ones are allowed (*see page 244*). Chocolate and vanilla are two perennial favorites. Rocombe Farm, who also produce frozen yogurts and sorbets, make around a dozen different ice creams, including lemon meringue and crunchies and cream, as well as specials such as Taste of Christmas.

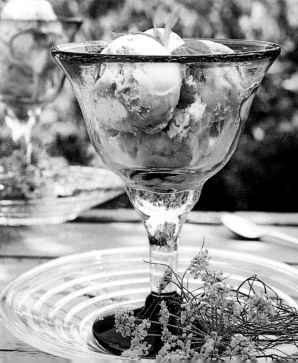

cream to organic, available in every store and through its nationwide home delivery service.

be prepared

Ready-cut vegetables are becoming available in supermarkets and, as with salad packs, washing in chlorine solutions is forbidden. Frozen organic peas, corn, spinach, carrots, lima beans, broccoli, and cauliflower are available from supermarkets and organic shops.

Cook's tip Frozen peas give winter stews and casseroles a lift – cook them and scatter over just before serving. They are also good stirred into rice and other grain dishes.

Focus on soy

Rich in proteins and nutritious oils, soy is one of the world's most perfect foods. Enjoyed for centuries in the East, it is becoming popular in the West as a healthy, versatile alternative to meat and dairy foods.

Soy beans are 35 percent protein. Just like animal protein, they contain all the essential amino acids that we need. They are high in fiber, and are a good source of vitamins and minerals. Soy beans are one of the few plant sources of the essential fatty acid alpha-linolenic acid and they also contain health-protecting phyto-estrogens – plant hormones that mimic estrogen. It is also thought that soy can have a direct effect on health. For example, eating soy beans is said to help combat diseases such as osteoporosis, certain cancers, and heart disease, and to alleviate menopausal symptoms.

versatility

As a food, soy is impressively versatile. Soy milk can be used in exactly the same way as cow's milk for all your cooking, as can soy cream. Tofu – soy bean curd – is crammed full of calcium and can be used in all kinds of ways as an alternative to meat. Various brands, found in most supermarkets, will smoke it, marinate it, spice it, or otherwise flavor it for you, making it even more convenient. Soy sauce and miso – both made from fermented soy beans – give a savory kick and are indispensable for all Eastern

dishes. Soy itself has become one of the world's most popular processing aids, and is used in an amazing variety of foods.

the gm specter

Since the advent of genetically modified (GM) strains, soy has rarely been out of the headlines. GM soy is grown extensively in the US and can be found in at least 60 percent of processed foods, from pizzas to ice cream, and in as much as 90 percent of animal feeds. Labeling laws do not require that GM derivatives such as lecithin derived from GM soy have to be declared on food labels. These laws also allow a GM tolerance threshold, which means that processed foods can contain up to one percent GM soy or other GM ingredients without legally having to declare this on the label. Animal feeds that contain GM ingredients do not have to be labeled at all. Organic foods, however, are guaranteed to have been made without any GM ingredients or derivatives and

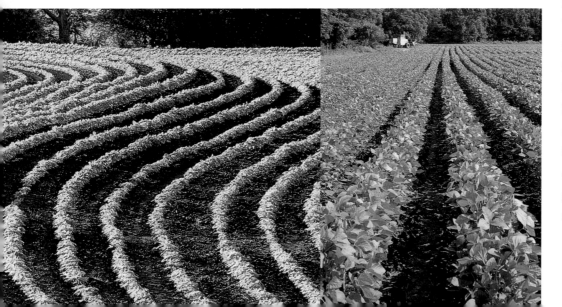

THE DIFFERENCES THAT COUNT

❖ Organic soy beans are grown without the use of artificial fertilizers and pesticides and as part of a mixed rotation

❖ The growing of GM soy beans is forbidden in organic farming

❖ Organic standards forbid the use of any GM soy or its derivatives in the growing or manufacture of any organic foods. By contrast, European labeling laws allow for up to one per cent contamination with GM soy in conventional processed foods before it needs to be declared on the label

❖ No GM soy (or its derivatives) are allowed in animal feeds approved for organic husbandry. It has been estimated that up to 90 percent of GM soy beans produced are used in the production of conventional animal feeds

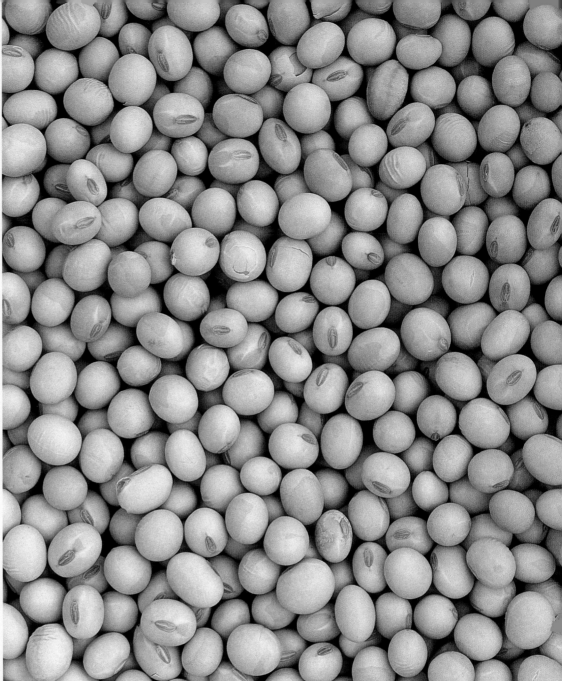

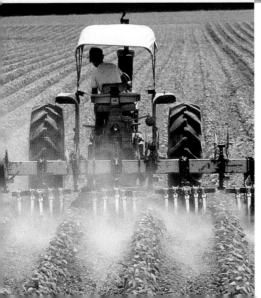

the use of both in organic animal feeds is also forbidden. Organic soy crops are not genetically engineered. Many organic soy product manufacturers are small concerns, who make organic tofu in the traditional way and their soy products in small batches.

Cook's tip To add a delicious depth of flavor to GM-free gravies, add a spoonful of organic tamari, shoyu, or soy sauce. These sauces are indispensable additions to your pantry essentials, as are other soy products, such as cubes of marinated, smoked, or fried tofu, which can be kept in the refrigerator. These are perfect for meat-free kebabs, stir-fries, oriental-style soups, noodle dishes, and vegetable casseroles.

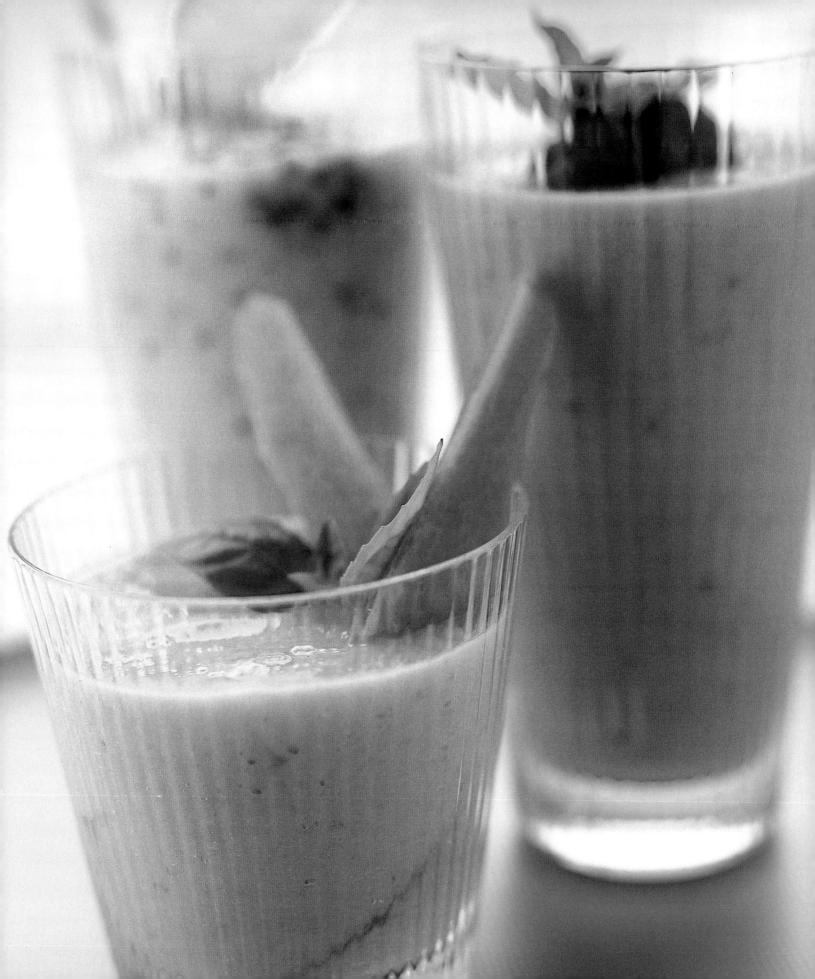

WHY DRINK
organic

For a healthy, happy lifestyle, what you drink is just as important as what you eat. Drinking organic is the natural choice for anyone who eats organic food, and, thanks to the wide range of drinks on offer, is easy to do.

Drinking organic offers you the same benefits as eating organic: a caring alternative and the confidence that you are choosing drinks you can trust. They are manufactured using ingredients produced without the barrage of harmful modern chemicals that crops such as conventional grapes, tea, coffee, grains, and sugar are all subjected to, with the disastrous implications this has had for human health and the environment.

Organic drinks contain no artificial additives or preservatives, and the use of genetically modified yeasts in brewing is prohibited. They are also produced mainly by small-scale, dedicated producers and manufacturers, which has particular benefits where wine is concerned (see page 112). Many organic teas and coffees are also fairly traded (see page 104). Converts, meanwhile, favor the cleaner flavors that many organic drinks and beverages have, and everyone susceptible to hangovers will vote for organic wines every time.

SPOILED BY CHOICE

As these pages also show, there is already a great selection of organic soft and alcoholic drinks. The organic drink and beverage industry is one of the fastest-growing sectors of the market. Hundreds of organic wines, organic beers, spirits, and champagnes, all kinds of health-giving organic juices and thirst-quenching organic soft drinks, not to mention a staggering range of organic teas, coffees, and herbal drinks, are all readily available and yours for the sipping.

ORGANIC CHEERS!

Every cup of organic tea or coffee, every bottle of organic apple juice, every delicious organic cocktail, and every glass of organic wine sipped on a summer's evening is a celebration of all that is good in life and of the heroes who are making a change for the better possible for all of us. Every sip is pure pleasure. Start today, raise your mug or glass and celebrate – the good life starts here.

Try a bottle of organic wine on your next visit to the supermarket

Ask for organic beers and at your local stores

Switch to organic coffee and tea – with organic milk, of course

Persuade your local restaurant to serve organic beverages

Seek advice from organic wine merchants

Heavenly
brews

The development of organic and fairly traded production of tea and coffee – the world's most popular beverages – provides inspiring examples of how environmental damage and welfare problems may be addressed.

Along with other commodity crops such as cocoa (*see page 95*) and bananas (*see page 68*), intensive production of tea and coffee causes devastation of the natural environment. By buying organic and fairly traded teas and coffees, we can help to reverse this and to improve the often appalling conditions for plantation workers – yet they cost almost nothing extra per cup.

Every story you read about organic or fair trade initiatives is inspirational. It means the use of toxic chemicals is reduced, wildlife is returning to landscapes and low-impact farming is providing long-term, sustainable solutions and security for all concerned. In India progressive working practices on some organic, Fairtrade tea plantations are providing new role models, especially for women.

on the slopes

Organic tea and coffee are generally grown in remote and isolated places, often at high altitudes. Organic tea is grown mainly in India, but also in Nepal and Sri Lanka (*see page 35*), while organic coffee (*see above right*) is grown in Latin America, East Africa, and exotic locations such as the highlands of Papua New Guinea and Sumatra. Organic coffee beans are predominantly arabica, which are the best-quality beans. Organic farms tend to be smaller than their non-organic counterparts, and self-sustaining, with tea and coffee grown as cash crops to raise money for medicines, education, and clothing. They are grown alongside other crops and animals that provide food, milk, and dung for fuel and soil fertility.

Growing practices include using mulches and a range of natural fertilizers, and planting shade plants and other plants and herbs that attract natural predators and beneficial insects.

initiatives

The fact that we can enjoy organic and fairly traded coffee today is thanks to heroic organizations such as Twin Trading. They have worked with marginalized, small-scale coffee farmers over the last 15 years to develop the Fairtrade supply chains (*see page 220*) on which successful brands such as Equal Exchange and Cafédirect depend.

Another inspirational initiative can be found in northern Peru. With increasing political stability in the area, farmers there that once grew coca – the cocaine-

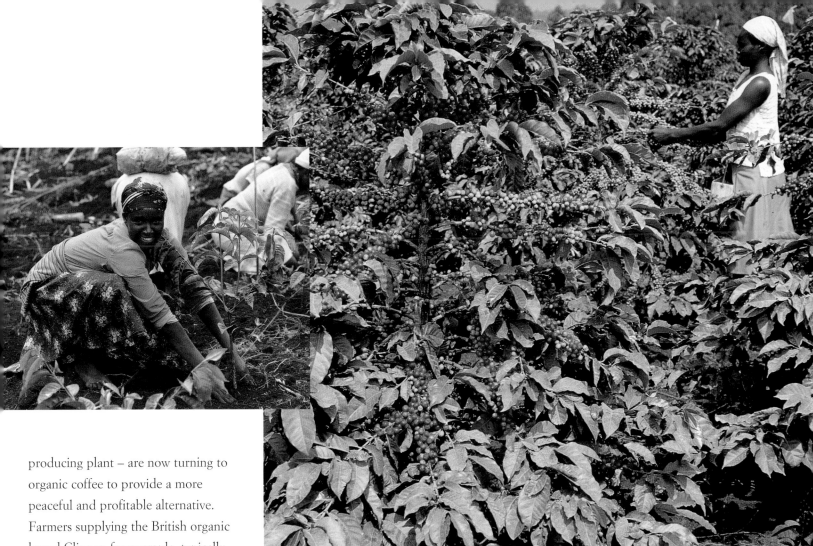

producing plant – are now turning to organic coffee to provide a more peaceful and profitable alternative. Farmers supplying the British organic brand Clipper, for example, typically farm 2.5–5 acres, growing coffee, cocoa, and a range of vegetables, including yuca, a staple carbohydrate in Peru. Every two acres yields around 1,760 lb (800 kg) of organic coffee, and earns farmers almost double the amount they used to receive from growing coca. Meanwhile their coffee beans are used in Clipper's instant organic coffee, on sale in British supermarkets.

options for all

Whatever your daily cup, be it tea, coffee or a calming herbal infusion, the organic option has something for everyone. Coffee may be bought as beans, ground beans, instant freeze-dried powder, or granules. Some large supermarkets and many smaller specialty markets are beginning to carry organic coffees. All the popular black and green teas are available, loose and in tea bags, plus a wide range of traditional and new ones, and exotic British organic spiced teas such as Hampstead Tea and Coffee's Biochai Masala, a blend of organic tea, ginger, cardamom, lemon grass, cloves, and black pepper. Organic herbal teas are another "must": chamomile and peppermint are perfect at the end of a meal. Lemon verbena tea is one of France's best-kept secrets and packs a fragrant lemon punch. There are more than 100 different herbal blends to try, including Ayurvedic organic herbal teas, Egyptian "kakade" (hibiscus) tea, and exotic and medicinal blends. All are made from certified organic herbs, are caffeine- and tannin-free, and are packed in bags that have not been treated with any chlorine.

The soft option

At those times when a cool, refreshing soft drink is the order of the day, it is good to know that your organic options now include everything your thirst could wish for.

Whatever your taste – sparkling or flat, herbal or fruity, traditional or new, canned or bottled – the organic choice is there for you, including an ever-increasing range of cordials and all the health-giving juices under the sun.

drink organic

All organic drinks are produced using certified organic ingredients and conform to organic processing standards. This means they are free from artificial flavorings and preservatives. Ascorbic acid (vitamin C) and tartaric acid (sodium tartrate, found naturally in grapes) are the only natural preservatives allowed. Although some organic soft drinks are healthier than other soft drinks, they are not necessarily lower in sugar. However, many organic manufacturers prefer using honey, apple juice, or agave syrup (a sweet syrup extracted from the leaves of the blue agave cactus) instead of sugar to sweeten drinks. As with all organic processed foods and drinks, the labels will tell you exactly what they contain, so you can decide for yourself.

Most soft drinks are simply water, sugar and flavorings. Organic soft drinks aim to do better. Whole Earth's canned organic cola contains lemon juice instead of phosphoric acid and real cola nut extract instead of caffeine to provide a natural lift. Organic apple juice and Mexican agave syrup, rather than refined white sugar, provide sweetness and a prolonged energy boost with just one-tenth of the glucose of conventional colas. And, instead of being laced with preservatives, Whole Earth's cola is pasteurized in the can.

bottled up

Bottled organic juices are the pure thing, squeezed from organically produced fruit and vegetables and carefully bottled to retain as many nutrients as possible. They serve as both food and drink and can be enjoyed throughout the day. Quality control is strict and many are produced by highly respected British specialist organic juicing companies such as Biotta, Rabenhorst, and Voekel. Once opened, bottled juices will keep in the refrigerator for a week or so. Mini-bottles – just the right size for packed lunches and children's lunch boxes – are also widely available.

Top tip Make fruit refreshers by diluting bottled fruit juices with sparkling mineral water, then adding a twist of organic lemon or orange.

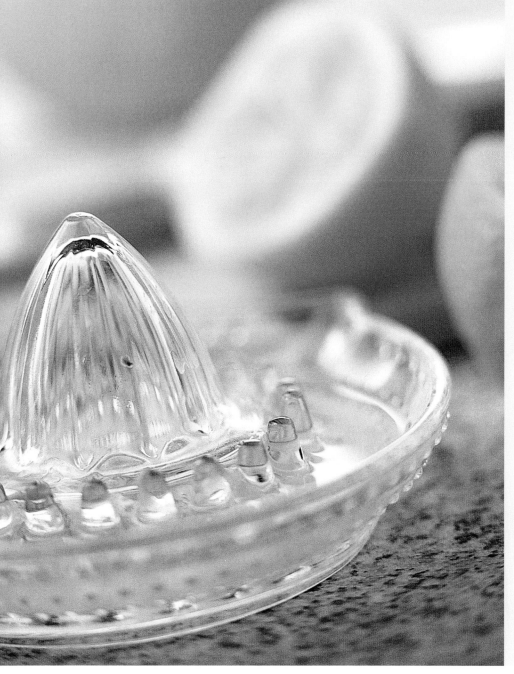

SQUEEZY DOES IT

Juicing has become one of the latest health crazes. Nothing is healthier or packs a more vital punch. To try them, head for the juice bars in organic supermarkets or, even better, buy a juicer – there are lots to choose from – and have fun experimenting at home:

❖ Try a blend of savory carrot and apple juices, with a dash of beet or celery, for a concentrated burst of vitamins

❖ Make fresh and fruity pick-me-ups by combining strawberries, kiwis, and any other soft fruit around

❖ Give your juices an extra zing and healthy goodness by adding fresh lemon juice or ginger

❖ Blend your own meal-in-a-glass smoothies, with bananas and organic yogurt or milk (or almond, rice, or soy milk for vegans), adding other soft fruits or pineapple according to availability and preference

apple juice

Organic apple juice is a popular choice and many commercial brands are available in supermarkets. Locally, look for organic apple juices from organic fruit growers at organic food markets and farmer's markets around the country. They are most often produced by the growers themselves and are excellent. They are often made from single varieties but can be found in made with combinations of apples. Each has its own characteristic flavor and sweetness profile, depending on the apple variety used to make it.

Top tip Serve organic apple juice at room temperature or lightly chilled. It is delicious as a base for fruit salads, punches and nonalcoholic fruit drinks, and used on muesli instead of milk.

Organics on the rocks

Such is the demand for organic alcoholic drinks, there is now an increasing range of organically produced spirits, beers, and hard ciders available from specialist suppliers and also from your local supermarket.

Just as with organic food, all organic alcoholic drinks are produced using certified organic ingredients – they contain no artificial additives, and no genetically modified ingredients or yeasts are used.

spirits

The production processes for organic spirits are on the whole no different than those used for conventional spirits, and although finding organic versions of some spirits can be difficult, the range is growing. There is an organic single malt whisky, for instance, distilled by Springbank from organic barley called Dà Mhìle, which is Gaelic for "2000". Vodka and gin are distilled to higher degrees of purity than whisky and the same basic rules apply. Organically produced raw materials, including the spices used for flavoring gin, are distilled in the standard way. Those to look out for include UK5 and Kentucky Rain vodkas and Juniper Green, a new all-organic London gin with organic botanical herbs sourced from all around the world – and remember the organic tonic. Organic cognac is produced using organic caramel, which is added to brandies to standardize the color and add flavor. Other organic spirits include calvados, an apple brandy made from distilled cider, and other grape brandies such as Italian grappa, as well as various fruit liqueurs.

beers & lagers

Demand for organic beers is booming – and not just from the specialist retailers. Many markets now offer a range of organic beers, and some organic specialists, such as Vintage Roots, even sell own-label versions. In addition to the British beers you can also find organically made German pilsner, dark and light wheat beers, lagers and a variety of Belgian types. Or try Cannabia, the first organic hemp beer, brewed in Germany, for something different. This burgeoning demand is tempered only by shortages of raw materials. Growing organic hops is not always easy, especially in coutnries like the UK with their unpredictable climate. Award-winning organic fruit grower and pioneer Peter Hall, based in Kent, is the UK's first certified organic hop producer, and his hops can be found in Brakspear's new organic beers such as Naturale. Organic hops are imported, however, from as far afield as New Zealand to supply the heavy

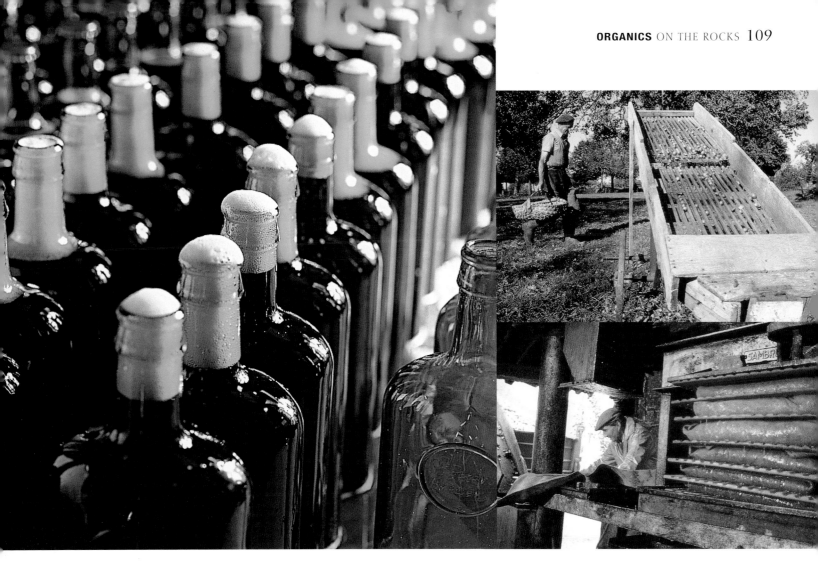

demand. Brewers have been impressed by the quality of organic hops, which offer great aroma and flavor, and impart a liveliness and zing to the beers. In the UK there are now ten organic brewers certified by the Soil Association, and more are sure to follow. The St. Peter's Brewery in England is one brewer that has recently added an organic beer to its range (*see above*). This beer is produced using locally malted barley and Kentish hops together with the latest innovations and quality control measures.

Top tip Pouring beer – especially bottle-conditioned beers containing sediment – needs attention. Tip the glass at a slight angle and pour the beer in gently down its side to avoid foaming, then bring the glass upright towards the end to give a small head if desired. If the beer contains sediment leave the last little bit in the bottle.

hard ciders

Organic hard cider production methods are much the same as those used to produce conventional hard ciders. However, the apples used to make organic hard ciders must come from organic orchards and certification bodies regulate the amounts of sulphur dioxide that the ciders may contain. Traditional farmhouse ciders may be made by pressing the apples with a "cheese" of straw (*see above*), and in that case the straw itself must also be organic. If sweeteners are added to the ciders, they must be organically produced too. Organic varieties in the UK include hard ciders from Aspall's, Dunkerton's, and Weston's. Delicious varieties are also produced, and sometimes imported, from Normandy, France.

From vine to wine

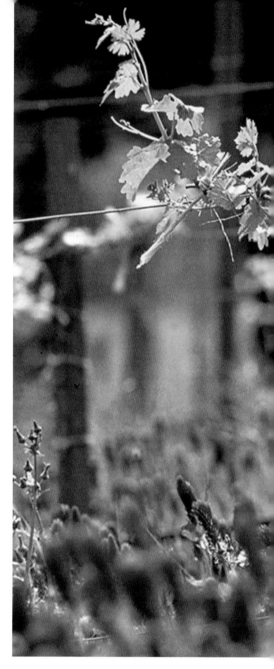

As the quality and range of organic wines continue to grow, buyers are finding that they have never had better choice, taste, and value.

These days wines seem to taste more and more alike. It is becoming harder to find wines of character that taste different and interesting. This is where organic wines score. They are made from organically grown grapes with minimum intervention in the winery. Organic producers work closely with the rhythms of nature (*see page 112*), and allow the grapes to speak for themselves. This can give organic wines a clear, pure flavor, and an individuality – the sense of coming from a particular place and time rather than some great amorphous wine lake.

fine wine

To find good organic wine, get to know the wines of different producers. Find names to follow – from a guidebook, to start with, or by experimenting and finding ones you like. Remember, wine-drinking is one of those happy activities where the only person you need to please is you. There are only two questions you have to ask yourself: "Do I like this wine?" and "Do I think it's worth the asking price?" (Those with sensitivities and allergies also need to ask themselves whether the wine agrees with them, but the chances are that if it is organic, it will.) Organic wines need not cost much more than their conventional counterparts. In all but the cheapest wines, the price differential is not generally very large, and you have the benefit of knowing that you are buying a top quality organic product.

Hot, dry climates make organic grape growing easier, so look out for southern French reds and Italian whites. Italian white wines in particular really appear to benefit from the organic approach; it seems to give them far more character and flavor than their conventionally grown counterparts. Given their ideal climate, it is surprising that so little organic wine is produced in Australia.

Top tip Look for the phrase "wine made from organically grown grapes" on wine labels, since there is currently no agreed European standard for "organic" wine.

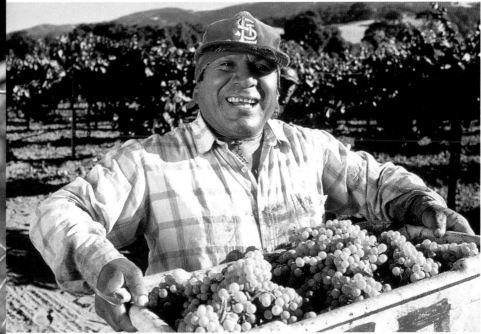

no hangover?

Compared to conventional wine, organic wine offers a great bonus: fewer allergic reactions and even, some say, less of a hangover the morning after. The prime hangover suspect is sulphur. Although notorious for causing allergic reactions in asthmatics, sulphur, in the form of sulphites, is a necessary part of the wine-making process. It protects the growing grapes from fungal attack, and preserves and stabilizes the finished wine. Sulphites form naturally during fermentation so no wine can ever be totally sulphite-free. Yet some wines contain extraordinarily high levels of sulphites, others next to none. Without accurate labeling information the simplest way to keep sulphur consumption in check is to drink organic, because the level set for sulphur in organic wine is lower than that for conventional wines. Specialist organic retailers can tell you which of their wines contain the least sulphur. These retailers can also show you files bulging with thank-you letters from customers who have been delighted to find that they can drink organic wines without suffering unpleasant side effects.

pass the port

Fortified organic wines such as port and sherry are also available, as are delicious nongrape organic wines such as ginger, blackcurrant, elderflower, elderberry, and apple. Most of these are produced in the UK, which may mean a slightly higher cost due to importation. Names to look out for include Broughton Pastures and Sedlescombe.

storage

Organic wines should be stored and served like any other. To keep wine, store it on its side so that the cork stays moist. Dry corks shrink and let air in, spoiling the wine. If the wine is unfiltered and has a deposit, stand it upright for a few hours before opening so the sediment has time to sink to the bottom of the bottle.

Focus on wine

Organic wine requires dedication and attention to detail all year round. This means that there is an emphasis on monitoring and caring for the vines, demanding great expertise.

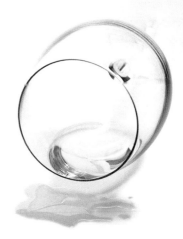

Organic vineyards often look and sound quite different to conventional ones. Most conventional vineyards are silent – insecticides kill pests and predators indiscriminately, and herbicides create scorched earth between the vines, giving the beneficial insects nowhere to live. By contrast, organic producers promote biodiversity by practiing companion planting – growing grasses and wild flowers with the vines – to encourage beneficial insects. The vineyards look beautiful all summer long and the air is alive with the hum and buzz of insects going about their business.

labor of love

Organic wines are sometimes more expensive to produce than conventional wines. Even though organic producers save on synthetic fertilizers and pesticides, the hands-on care organic vines demand means that more is spent on labor. Often organic producers insist on lower yields – this means they produce fewer bottles per acre, but of improved flavor and concentration. Rather than using artificial fertilizers, organic producers often grow "green manure" crops (*see page 154*) between vine rows to fix essential nutrients, and use composted materials including grape skins and seeds saved from the previous year's harvest to build up soil fertility – perfect recycling. This approach is typified by Fetzer of California, one of the world's largest growers of organic grapes, who compost over 10,000 tons of grape skins and seeds each year. Fetzer also proves that large companies can be environmentally responsible too. Since the mid-1980s it has been at the cutting edge of organic farming techniques and sustainable business practices, recycling tons of waste paper, wine cartons, and glass, and using wax seals on their bottles instead of lead capsules.

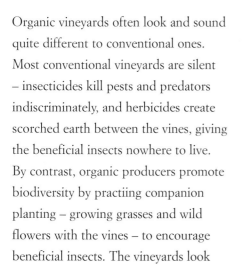

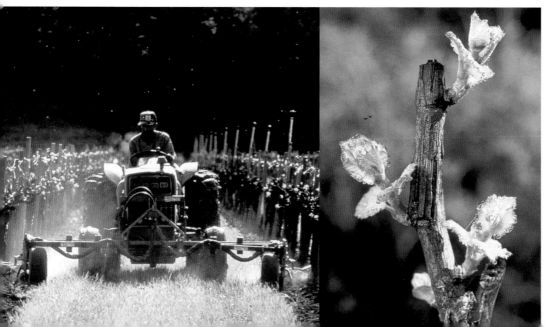

THE DIFFERENCES THAT COUNT

✤ The use of artificial fertilizers, insecticides and herbicides in organic vineyards is not permitted

✤ Organic grape producers promote biodiversity by planting flowers and plants between the vines to attract beneficial predatory insects

✤ The production of organic grapes is labor-intensive and relies on hands-on care and expertise

✤ Soil fertility is enhanced by growing "green manure" crops

✤ Organic producers take an active approach to recycling by composting grape skins and seeds from the previous year's crop

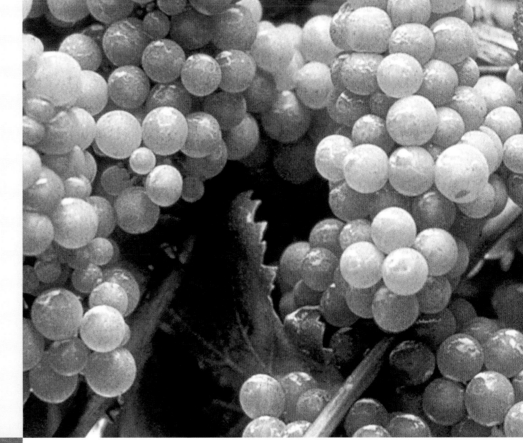

wine skills

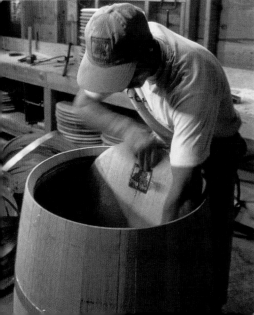

Although organic certification guarantees that the grapes used to produce organic wines have been grown according to organic standards, this is no guarantee of better quality. Organic producers need, if anything, to be better wine-makers than those who do it the chemical way. Without the back-up of an arsenal of chemicals, they need to be very observant, sensitive and knowledgeable. The key to producing good wine is letting it speak for itself. Sometimes this can be tough for wine-makers who have a preconceived idea of how they want their wines to smell and taste, but this is the way organic producers make wines that buyers seek out time after time for their character and individuality.

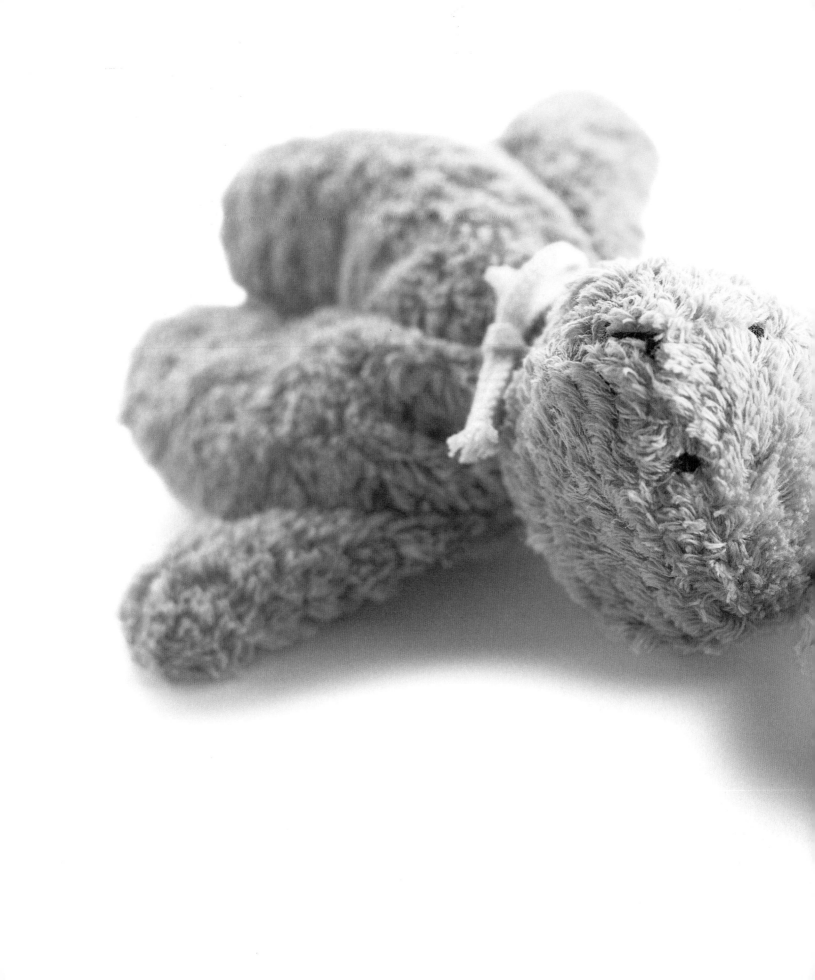

organic
BABY CARE

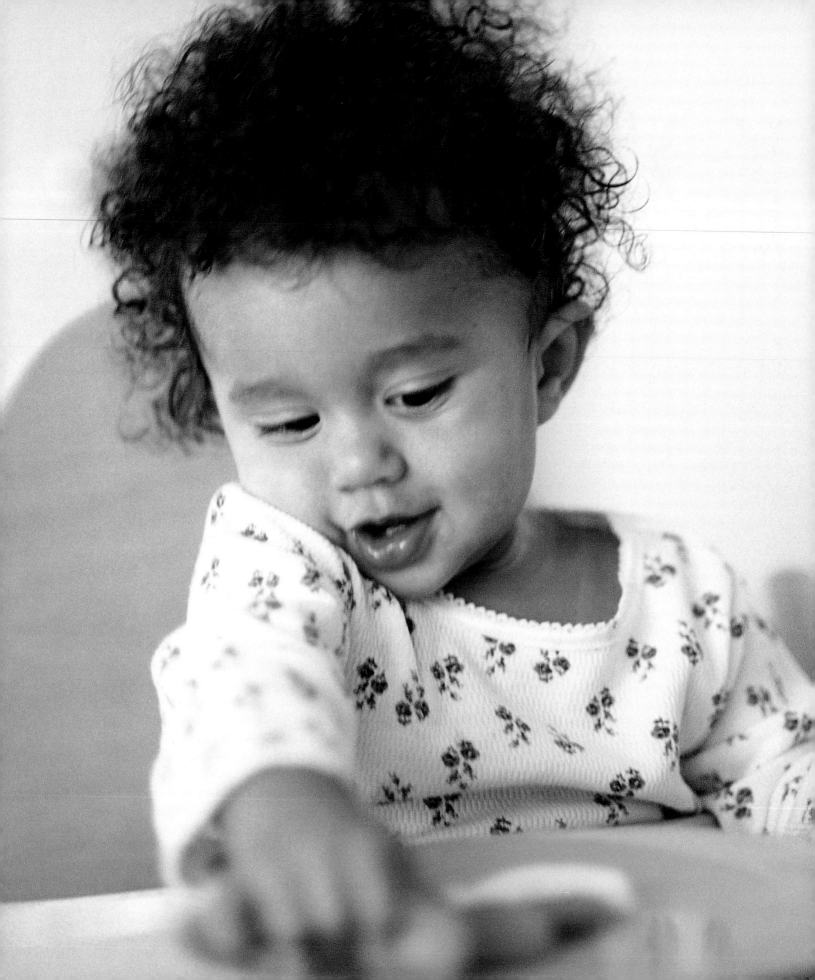

WHY ORGANIC baby care

The ever-increasing availability of organic foods and products means that organic parenting is now a reality. Parents today have the chance to offer their children the best possible organic start in life.

We all want the best for our children, and it is natural for us to want to protect and nurture them as well as possible. Providing your baby with high-quality nourishment and a secure environment in which to grow is a huge responsibility. As many thousands of parents will testify, it is becoming increasingly clear that an organic approach is the best way to feed and care for your baby.

TOXIC LEGACY OR HEALTHY FUTURE?

The dangers that threaten us all from toxic chemicals loom even larger for our babies and children. In the food that you feed them, the products you use to bathe and soothe them, and the diapers and clothes in which you wrap them, you are unwittingly in danger of exposing them to a potentially harmful cocktail of toxic chemicals. It is in the critical stages of growth and development that they are most susceptible to the dangers posed by pollutants.

Growing evidence suggests that what children eat and how they are cared for during the early stages of their lives has a direct and lasting effect on their later health and development. Many health problems associated with children may be due to the effects of toxins on their vulnerable immune systems, and exposure to chemicals in food and consumer goods has been linked directly to susceptibility to illness and diseases in later life.

A QUESTION OF CHOICE

If choosing the organic option for our babies and children is an investment in their present and future health and happiness, then the availability of organic foods and baby products means that this choice is now easy to make. And what better time is there, too, than when we start to consider the well-being of our children and our role as parents, for us to make positive choices about our own diet and lives?

Feed your baby or toddler with pure organic foods

Soothe your baby's skin with natural products

Wrap your baby in soft, natural, toxin-free organic fabrics

Tuck your baby into warm organic bedding at night

A spoonful of goodness

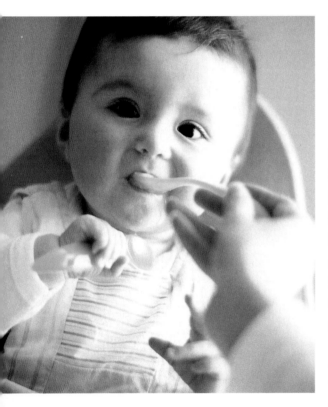

It is never too early to start. Many parents are finding that choosing healthy organic food is best for their baby.

When it comes to protecting your baby by choosing organic food, you can never start too early. Just as an organic farmer will prepare the seeds and soil to provide the best chances for a strong and healthy crop, so parents can ensure the optimum health of themselves and their offspring by eating organic prior to conception. Pre-conception programs that include following a diet of organic wholefoods have helped many couples worldwide conceive healthy babies born after healthy pregnancies. This is an important time when food quality should not be compromised.

feeding for two

The familiar warnings about the harmful effects of smoking, drinking alcohol, or taking drugs during pregnancy all clearly point to the link between a mother's lifestyle and the health of her developing baby. Although the uterus would seem the safest environment in which a baby can grow, it is while he or she is there that any toxins in your food may have an effect. Evidence suggests that chemicals used in nonorganic food production can affect the development of babies in the uterus and possibly lead to lowered immunity and health problems later in life. By eating organic foods, you can help to protect your baby.

breast-feeding

Breast-feeding is the most natural and wholesome way of feeding your baby because of the key nutritional elements in breast milk. It contains natural fatty acids and antibodies that can reduce the risk of infection and improve immunity. Regrettably, the presence of traces of

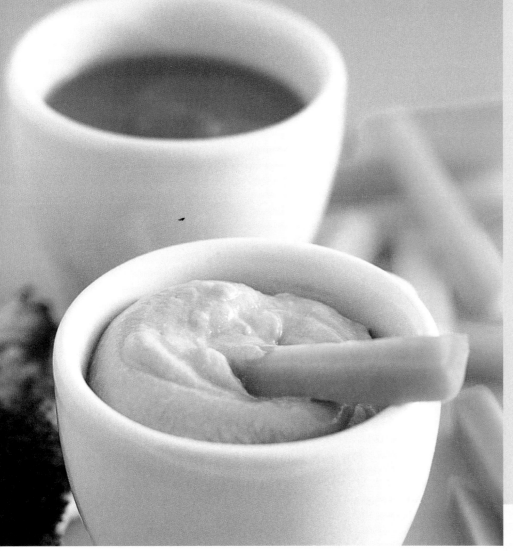

THE DIFFERENCES THAT COUNT

✤ Eating organic food during your pregnancy helps to avoid passing potential toxins to your baby while he or she is in the uterus

✤ The breast milk of mothers who eat organic foods that have no pesticide inputs is likely to contain less pesticide residues than the breast milk of those who eat food from agrochemical farming

✤ Only organic baby foods are certified to contain ingredients that are grown without any artificial fertilizers, pesticides, fungicides, growth hormones, and antibiotics

✤ Organic baby foods come with a guarantee that genetically modified organisms (GMOs) have not been used in any ingredient

artificial chemicals in breast milk is unavoidable. Choosing to eat organic foods yourself is likely to help reduce the levels of these.

formulas

When, for whatever reason, breast-feeding is not possible, baby milks and formulas are available, which are made from cow's milk that has been technically modified to replicate, as far as is possible, the complex and unique nutritional profile of breast milk. There are several brands of organic formula milks sold in supermarkets, health shops, and by mail order, providing a range of infant milks for newborns and follow-on milks for those over six months old.

spooning it in

While there is no doubt that the best and most economical way to feed your baby organic foods is to make your own, using preprepared versions only as a back up,

A spoonful of goodness

organic preprepared baby foods offer a useful combination of convenience and peace of mind. No surprise, then, that organic baby food is the fastest-growing sector of the organic food industry and over one third of all baby foods sold in the UK, for example, are organic. All baby foods are covered by legislation that bans the use of colorings, artificial sweeteners, preservatives, and added salt. But only organic baby foods are guaranteed free of ingredients grown with agrochemicals that may turn up as residues in their conventional

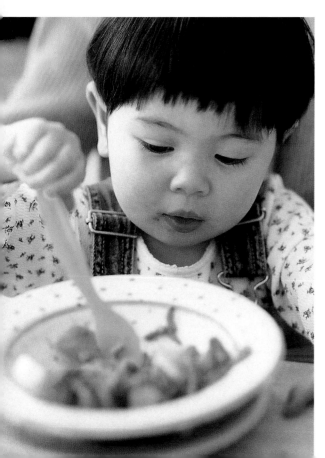

counterparts. Organic baby foods are also leading the way in introducing new high-quality, ingredients into the recipes and using clearer labeling information.

delicate bodies

The immaturity of babies' organs and body systems means that they are highly susceptible to the effects of toxins. Babies and young children also have a high potential exposure to toxins due to the large volumes and limited range of foods they eat. Compared to their body weight, they eat far more food than older children or adults, and the types of food they eat are limited to milk, fruit, and vegetables – precisely those foods in which residues are most often detected. This all means that you cannot afford to compromise on what you feed your baby.

Es & GMOs

Although the use of E-number additives is prohibited in all baby foods, they are present in a variety of nonorganic family foods that might find their way into your baby's diet. Hot dogs, for example, are often used as a child moves into the toddler stage. But the average hot dog contains over 7 nonfood additives, and

some contain up to 15. Organic standards prohibit the use of most of these, so choosing organic is preferable. Many parents are concerned about the use of baby food ingredients that may have been genetically modified (*see page 30*). If the fears that some scientists have over genetically modified foods are realized, babies and young children may be the first to suffer because the immaturity of their immune, digestive, and other body systems makes them more vulnerable.

buying organic

Organic baby food represents the cost of producing food you can trust. The good news is that increased demand and production means more affordable prices. Organic baby foods are now widely available through a variety of retailers and there are many brands to choose from. There is also a wide variety of foods to consider – vegetarian and nonvegetarian, meals, cereals, and baby pasta, drinks and juices, desserts, and yogurts. But be sure to survey the label carefully – it is strongly recommended that baby food should not contain added sugar, even if it is organic. Some organic baby food brands also use small amounts of nonorganic ingredients.

the producers

THE CHOICE IS YOURS

There is an ever-growing range of organic baby foods available. Baby Organix (*see above*) paved the way in the UK in 1992. Since then, Hipp from Germany and Olvarit from Nutricia in Holland have joined in. The Boots chain, in the UK, sells its own range and some supermarkets are following suit. Simply Organic of the UK, Babynat of France, and Eco-Baby of Holland are all organic and are in many health food shops and supermarkets.

PIONEERING SPIRIT

Baby Organix (*see above*) is the pioneering brand that helped to set up the organic baby food market in the UK.

It was launched in 1992 by mothers Lizzie Vann and Jane Dick, who set out to revolutionize baby foods by making pure baby foods that taste of real food, using ingredients you would find in your kitchen rather than industrial processing aids. The company is committed to organic farming and works closely with the organic farms responsible for supplying the produce that goes into its baby foods. This ensures that the company's products are made using only the highest-quality ingredients, which are listed in percentages on the side of the jars. Subsequently Lizzie has also launched Organix Favourites, a range of high-quality organic foods for older children. All the Organix foods contain no fillers, milk powders, added sugars, emulsifiers, or flavorings.

Organic baby food is a sure way of giving your child the very best start in life – an introduction to the pleasures and benefits of eating well.

LIZZIE VANN, FOUNDER, THE ORGANIX CHILDREN'S FOOD COMPANY

Wrapped in organics

Having chosen to feed your baby organic foods, the natural next step is to ensure that your baby care products, bedding, and even toys are as safe and natural as they can be.

The speed at which the range of organic baby care products is growing means that demand is rising and prices are falling. This is good news for all parents who want the best for their babies.

diapers

A diaper is the one item of clothing your baby spends the most time in, so it is important to choose the right type. In recent years many parents have moved away from traditional cloth diapers, since disposables seem to offer a quicker, more convenient option. However, governments and environmentalists are becoming increasingly concerned about the effects of disposable diapers on both health and the environment. As well as chemical additives, including bleaches, lotions, plastics, and perfumes, most disposable diapers contain a layer of super-absorbent gel in the fluff pulp. Small beads of this gel can escape from the diaper and come in contact with a baby's skin or even the mouth.

Furthermore, disposables are non-biodegradable. In the UK, they make up more than four percent of total household waste, but cannot be flushed or composted, and they are dumped in landfills where they can take 200 years to decompose. During your baby's diaper-wearing lifetime you will use roughly 5,500 diapers – that's an estimated cost of over $1500 to you, and an environmental cost of more than 2,755 lb (1,250 kg) of nonbiodegradable waste.

A better choice for your baby's health and the environment is to use cloth diapers. There are plenty of varieties to choose from, and diaper laundry services in most areas of the US for those who do not have time to cope with the added laundry. If you can find them, organic cotton diapers are the best option. Many stores in the UK have a selection of washable diapers, and they are also available from mail-order companies. A list of companies supplying them is available in the organic directory at the back of this book. You can also check with local mothering organizations and magazines for their lists of cloth diaper companies who, for a flat weekly fee (usually at around the same price as a week's supply of disposable diapers), will provide you with a supply of diapers and pick up your dirty ones every week. Some laundering services use eco-

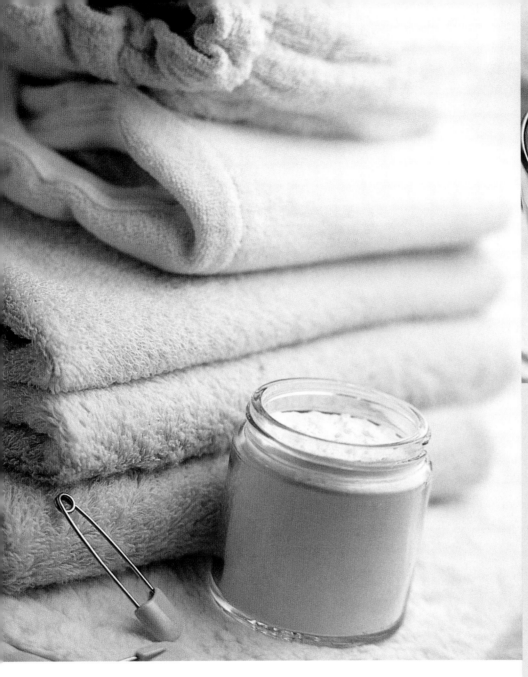

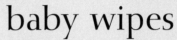

baby wipes

Most commercial baby wipes for your baby's bottom contain alcohol or other ingredients that can irritate a baby's skin. The best baby wipe for both your baby and the environment is a washable wipe, preferably made from organic or undyed cotton. Buy a dozen or so washable wipes, available from most cloth diaper companies, and use them with a homemade wipe solution or water. The following recipe can be used to make an effective, soothing wipe:

3¹/₂ tbsp (50 ml) distilled water
1 tbsp (15 ml) vinegar
2 tbsp (30 ml) aloe vera gel
1 tbsp (15 ml) calendula oil
1 drop lavender essential oil
1 drop tea tree essential oil

The vinegar and essential oils will act as a preservative, so you can store the solution for up to six weeks.

friendly laundry detergents. If you do choose disposables, try to find the most healthy and environmentally friendly varieties that can be found at many specialty markets.

In the US several brands of eco-friendly diaper are available from health shops, by mail order or in pharmacies. Tushies disposables, produced here in the US, are free of chemical gels, latex,

dyes, and perfumes. Weenees, an Australian diaper, has a reusable outer pant with a disposable inner pad. These pads are free from plastic, but do contain an absorbent chemical gel. Another variation is Moltex Öko, a disposable diaper from Germany that uses recycled pulp in its construction and is unbleached, but also uses a chemical gel for added absorbency.

Wrapped in organics

diaper rash

Most babies will get diaper rash at some time. Usually it is caused by prolonged contact with soiled diapers, but it may also be a symptom of teething, or of a reaction to new foods or to detergents, perfumes, or other chemicals used in some disposable diapers, wipes, or lotions. Even if you use super-absorbent disposables they still need to be changed frequently to help prevent diaper rash. There are natural products that may help protect against diaper rash by creating a barrier between your baby's skin and urine, and powders can help prevent rashes. Avoid powders containing cosmetic talcum powder, since the fine particles can get into babies' lungs. Instead, use a natural powder made from cornstarch or arrowroot. Perhaps the best cure for diaper rash is fresh air, so let your baby go without a diaper as often as you can.

soaps

Your new baby's skin requires very little more than water for the first few weeks. There is no need to interfere with a baby's perfect skin as it has very few chances to get dirty. Once you do need to start using soap, use a moisturizing natural olive oil soap sparingly and rinse it off well. When buying baby care products bear in mind that the skin absorbs much of what is put on it, so check the list of ingredients carefully and avoid anything artificial. If organic ingredients are used the products do tend to work out more expensive, but remember – a little goes a long way. There are currently no regulations covering what can legally be certified as "organic" toiletries but in the UK, for example, companies such as Green People, Neal's Yard, and Weleda are working alongside the Soil Association to set regulations and standards.

baby clothes

Natural fibers will allow your baby's skin to breathe. The best fabrics to dress your baby in are cotton, wool, or silk – preferably organic (*see page 199*). Conventional cotton is one of the crops most heavily treated with artificial pesticides, and in some countries cotton has also been genetically engineered or treated with formaldehyde, a known carcinogen. Only wool from organically reared sheep is guaranteed to have not been dipped in organophosphates.

By avoiding conventionally produced clothing you may be able to help alleviate many allergic and asthmatic symptoms as well as skin problems in your child. There are quite a few companies, here in the US, that offer organic baby clothing. Many use as many organic materials as possible such as organic cotton and organic dyes. Organic clothes are usually more expensive than their conventional equivalents, so you may prefer to choose only a few items of organic clothing.

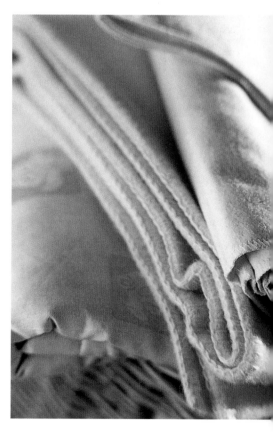

If you do, concentrate on those that your baby will wear next to the skin, such as undershirts and onesies. If you do not buy organic cotton or woolen clothing, try to at least use only those that are licensed under American or other European regulatory organizations. Clothing with these certificates has been tested for chemical processing and will be free of formaldehyde, waxes, bleaches, and other harmful chemicals.

bedding

Most new conventional cot mattresses will have been treated with fire- and water-retardant chemicals. These chemicals may cause respiratory problems and skin allergies. Organic cotton and wool mattresses for cots are available from a variety of mail order companies and, for a little more money, offer more peace of mind. A more affordable alternative might be a natural futon, that is stuffed with organic cotton or wool. If you decide to buy a new conventional mattress, try to avoid one filled with polyurethane foam and also be sure to allow it to "off-gas" in a well-ventilated room for several days before allowing your baby to sleep on it. Try to make sure that what is closest to your baby's skin is organic or untreated fabric. Organic or untreated cotton sheets, for example, and wool blankets are quite easy to find through mail order companies and some retailers (*see pages 237 and 241*).

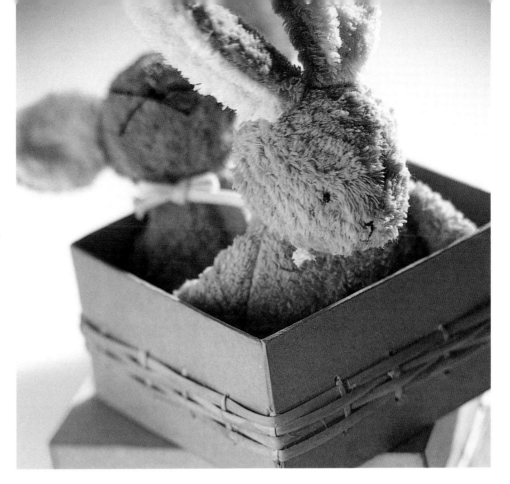

accessories

Even getting out and about with your baby can be an organic experience, thanks to the range of strollers, baby slings, and even car seats made using organic fabrics that are available. The price of some of these larger items is substantial, but a smaller item such as a baby sling requires only a relatively minor investment. Lamb skins are a very popular item on most new parents' shopping lists, and those made from organically reared sheep are available. With the ban on the use of organophosphate dips still only voluntary, it is important to ensure that your baby's lamb skin does not come from a sheep that has been exposed to

these chemicals. Organic lamb skins will have been naturally tanned using mimosa rather than by synthetic tanning methods.

toys

One of the rewards of going organic is knowing that even the toys you give your baby are free of harmful chemicals. Toys are the things your baby is most likely to suck or chew, so it is wise to know what they are made of. Soft PVC toys contain chemicals that may be harmful. Many manufacturers have pledged to stop making toys with PVC but there is, as yet, no ban in the US. The best toys are those made using natural materials, such as natural wooden toys and organic cotton animals, which make great playmates.

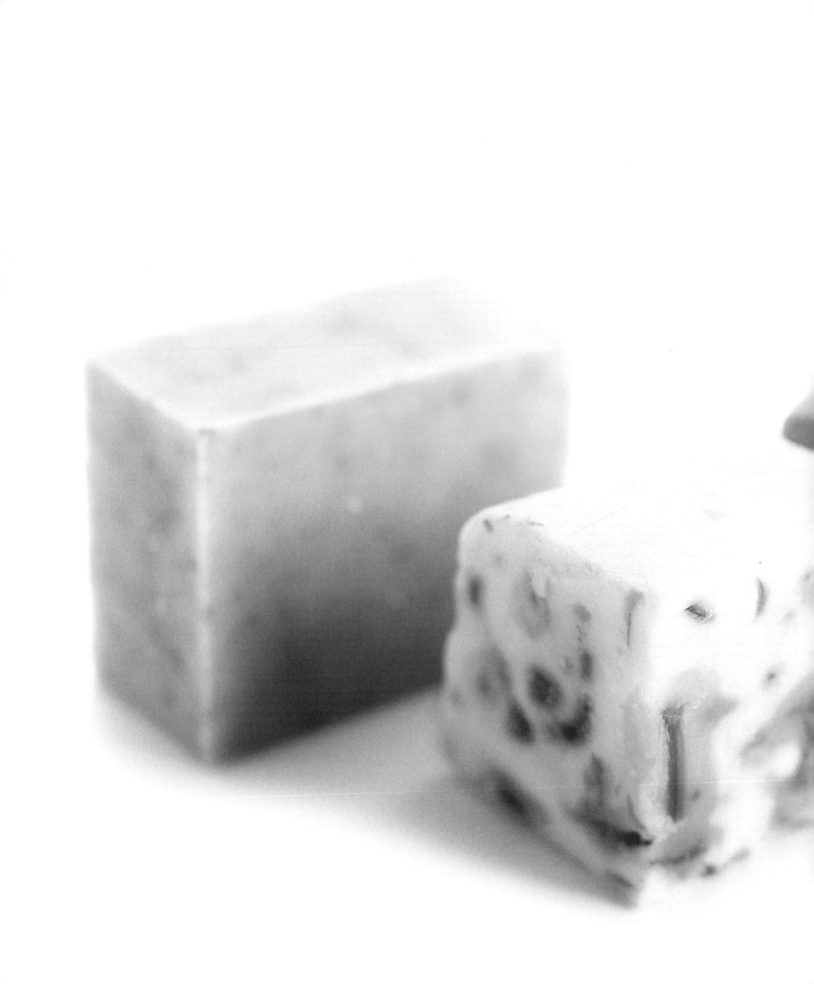

organic

HEALTH & BEAUTY

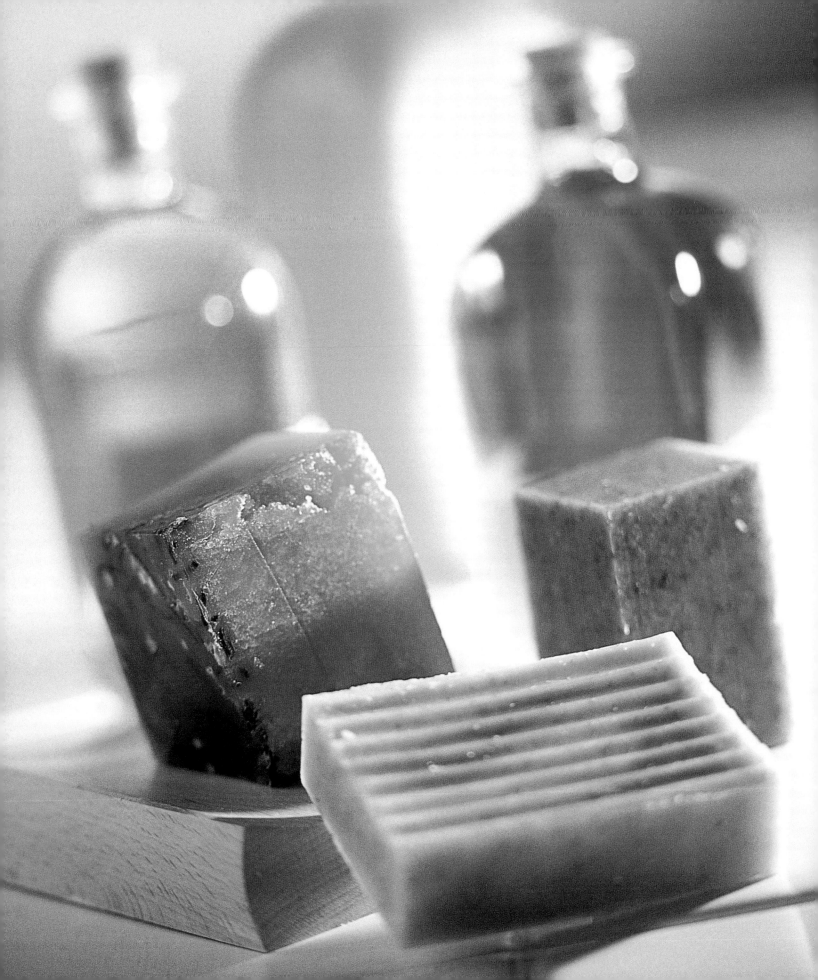

WHY GO
organic

Once you have started eating organic food, it is only a matter of time before you will think about the cosmetics you put on your skin – which are, after all, "skin foods" – and your approach to health and well-being.

When it comes to beauty rituals like skin care, make-up, and bathing, there is one very good reason for taking a more natural approach – because the skin drinks in what you apply to it. If you have ever wondered where a body lotion goes when you massage it in, the answer is: some evaporates and some is absorbed not only into your skin, but also into the bloodstream. If you avoid artificial chemicals in your daily diet, the logical next step is to "green" your beauty regime. And if you are concerned not only about your own health but that of the environment, it makes sense to seek out cosmetics that are sustainably produced – avoiding, for instance, ingredients such as mineral oil and petrolatum, which are nonrenewable resources.

INVESTIGATE ALTERNATIVES

Food for thought, meanwhile, is the fact that many medicines are produced by the very same companies that make pesticides, herbicides, and other agrochemicals. When we are critically ill, those medicines can be lifesavers. But many of us reach for painkillers, sleeping pills, or even cough medicines on a daily basis when there are excellent nature-based alternatives that people used for centuries before modern medicines were developed.

TAKE CONTROL OF YOUR HEALTH

For many people, just taking a more active approach to health – minimizing stress, getting enough exercise and eating plenty of fresh, wholesome, organic food – has the biggest effect of all, making history of many of the day-to-day health issues that have us lining up to see the doctor. And an added effect of eating organically is simply becoming more aware of food's impact on the body and mind – both positive and negative. This should make it easier for us to take charge of our own health instead of relying on those over-the-counter or prescribed medicines, and taking up so much of our valuable time at the doctor's.

Become a label reader and avoid products with long lists of ingredients

Discover complementary therapies to promote optimum health

Let food be your medicine by eating a balanced diet based on organic fruit, vegetables, grains, and legumes

Make simple cosmetics at home using fresh organic ingredients

A dose of good

When you are ill, it is all too easy to reach for the pills. A more positive approach is to think "holistically" about your health – how your diet, lifestyle, and healthcare choices can promote your well-being.

Most drugs are synthetic chemicals. Some may contain active plant elements, but it is usually cheaper to synthesize them in a laboratory. This also "standardizes" medicines, so that drugs manufacturers can be certain of an exact dose every time. In nature the seasons, the weather and the maturity of a plant are all variables that can potentially alter a plant's potency.

popping pills

Today, we have become used to "a pill for every ill" – quick-fix solutions to health problems that enable us to be back at our desks, or caring for our families, as quickly as possible. As a result, drugs are massively over-prescribed – with potentially disastrous effects. When antibiotics were first introduced, for instance, they were hailed as a miracle, saving literally millions of lives. But their over-use is leading to ever more virulent "superbugs", which threaten us with spiraling epidemics and unknown ills. In many cases doctors are merely responding to patients' demands for some kind of prescription when they come to the doctor's office, even for a flu or a cold – both viruses for which antibiotics are entirely ineffective.

well-being

Organic living takes a more positive, proactive approach to health. True health is not just the absence of illness, but a feeling of energy and vitality that comes from taking a "holistic" approach to our body, mind, and lifestyle. Part of this can be achieved through diet: eating three balanced meals a day and minimizing your intake of alcohol, caffeine, and unhealthy snacks. Another vital element in this holistic approach is stress reduction: finding ways of slowing down in a speeded-up world. The reason for this is not only so that we sail through life more calmly and capably without snapping at everyone around us, but also because evidence is emerging of a link between our state of mind and the health of our bodies.

Research suggests that stressed people are more vulnerable to illness – from minor ailments like colds right through to cancer. Today, the concept of "psycho-neuroimmunology" – in simple terms, how the mind affects our physical state – has gained wide acceptance. So it is absolutely vital to find ways to switch off and relax. There is no doctor's prescription for this, and the method will be different for each of us, whether it be yoga, a daily walk, massage, or playing the piano. However, if the activity is aerobic – such as swimming or running – you get a double benefit, giving your heart a workout while you are de-stressing. Also, the healing power of sleep should also not beunderestimated.

medicine

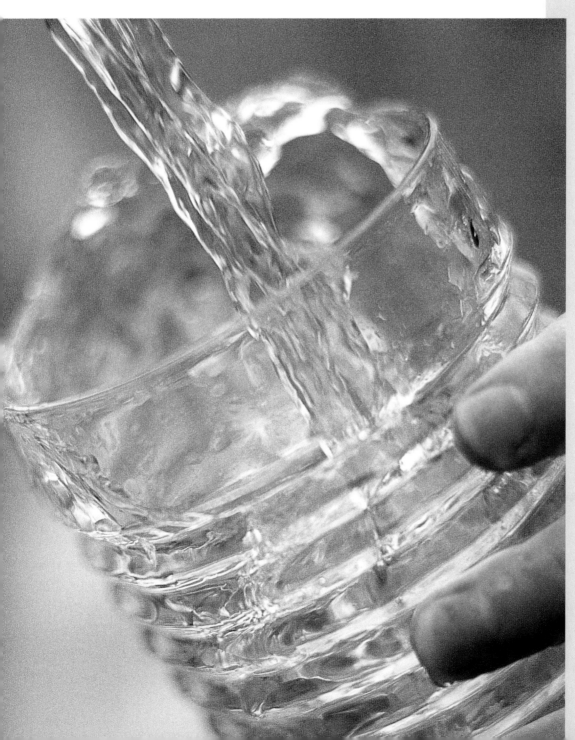

THE IMPORTANCE OF WATER

Drinking enough water is often underestimated or written off as merely a supermodel's eccentricity – they all swear by it, insisting it delivers clearer skin and a natural "glow". Enough water – 1.5 litres a day, preferably mineral water or filtered – does more than keep the body's system flushed and functioning, but helps our brain, too. If you have ever experienced an uncomfortably dry mouth – having to speak in public, perhaps – then it is worth thinking about the fact that your brain, too, is suffering from the same dehydration. Keeping well-hydrated makes it easier to think, and when we can think clearly, we feel less stressed. These "positive spirals" are what we should all be aiming for in the quest for better health.

A dose of good medicine

No matter how well we eat or how regularly we exercise, we all become ill at some time. For minor ailments and chronic conditions, it is worth considering a complementary approach (*see right*). (In the case of an accident or emergency, the emergency room of your local hospital should still be your first stop.) Today, many forms of complementary medicine are becoming integrated into mainstream medicine. Homeopathy and acupuncture, in particular, are being studied by an increasing number of conventional doctors. Complementary medicine actively seeks to promote health, even when we are not ill. In the case of Traditional Chinese Medicine (TCM), acupuncture or seasonal "tonics" are encouraged to maintain optimum health all year round.

detoxification

If you are worried about the toxins going into your body, you are probably also worried about the toxins that are already stored there. In fact, most of us have a frightening array of chemicals in our systems; in research, individuals have shown levels of chemicals which have long since been banned. Can detoxing get rid of them? Up to a point. Experts such as Dr. Udo Erasmus believe that eating a healthy balance of "good" fats and oils can help to maintain healthy liver function, flushing toxins from the system, whereas "trans-fats" – present in hydrogenated fats and oils (which are actually banned in organic production) – interfere with the liver's ability to detox.

These "good" oils, or essential fatty acids (EFAs), are found in oily fish, evening primrose oil, or, for ease, a pre-mixed blend of what are known as omega 6 and omega 3 EFAs, which are also available organically (*see page 95*).

A nutritional advisor at your health food store should be able to give you more information. If you are healthy and do not have abnormal blood pressure, heart problems, or diabetes, an occasional one-day fast or a few days of detoxing – mainly on fresh organic juices and raw vegetables – can also help cleanse your system, particularly in tandem with a program of skin-brushing. However, some toxins may remain in your system forever so, rather than be paranoid about the past, aim to minimize your exposure in every area of your life from now on.

treatments

Finding a drug-free way to stay healthy is important – not just to minimize our exposure to chemicals, but as a positive step towards well-being. But each of us is an individual; what works for your best friend may not be the perfect solution for you. Selection requires an element of trial and error, so do not give up on complementary medicine just because one technique does not work for you. In many cases, these therapies also cost money, requiring us to prioritize optimum health above, say, a long-haul holiday or a new car – choices that only we can make for ourselves.

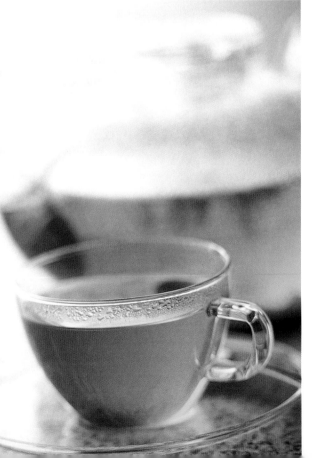

COMPLEMENTARY OPTIONS

Here are some of the most easily accessible therapies that you could try:

❖ **Acupuncture** – the insertion of fine needles (painlessly, in most cases) into the body's "energy channels", to balance energies and restore health and vitality.

❖ **Aromatherapy** – involves massages with scented oils to relax the mind and body. Its de-stressing effects have become so widely acknowledged that it is being used in hospitals and other medical institutions.

❖ **Flower Remedies** – the use of healing essences, distilled from flowers.

❖ **Herbalism** – the use of herbs to treat illnesses. Herbalism was originally based on herbs grown in the West, but has since expanded to include the use of herbs from around the world.

❖ **Homeopathy** – the use of minute amounts of natural substances to treat mind and body imbalances.

❖ **Naturopathy** – can be a combination of diet, osteopathy, and hydrotherapy (water therapy), used to treat illness and boost good health. It is particularly effective for some chronic illnesses such as premenstrual tension and irritable bowel syndrome.

❖ **Reflexology** – the pressure-point massage of energy points on the feet that relate to different organs in the body.

❖ **Traditional Chinese Medicine** – the prescription of Chinese herbs, based on a different system of diagnosis and health analysis to that of Western doctors. The herbs can be boiled to make a "tea" at home, or, in some cases, taken in the form of small, black, licorice-based pills.

A NATURAL MEDICINE CABINET

Instead of reaching for an over-the-counter remedy, why not try the alternatives below? These are more natural than anything you will find in a pharmacy. If symptoms persist, consult your doctor or natural health practitioner.

❖ **Aloe vera** may help to heal minor burns and cuts and to soothe sunburn. You can squeeze the juice directly from the leaf of the plant, or use an over-the-counter cream or gel.

❖ **Arnica** gel or ointment is a remedy for strained and aching muscles. Homeopathic arnica is good to have in your medicine cabinet to take after trauma or shock, and for swift wound-healing.

❖ **Chamomile** tea is considered good for indigestion, anxiety, insomnia, headaches, and premenstrual symptoms.

❖ **Clove** oil is a highly effective natural painkiller, especially for toothache.

❖ **Echinacea** is an immune stimulant. It is useful if you are feeling run-down, and is available as a herb, in capsules or as an easy-to-take tincture.

❖ **Eucalyptus** oil opens up breathing passages to relieve colds: dilute a few drops in hot water for a steam inhalation, or add a few drops to a hot bath.

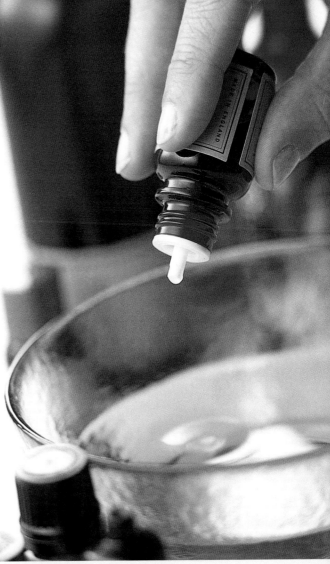

❖ **Feverfew and white willow bark** are natural painkillers. You can sometimes find them mixed together in capsules.

❖ **Lavender** essential oil may help ease anxiety, insomnia and minor burns: use in a diffuser or add to a bath. (Lavender and tea-tree essential oils are the only ones that can be used neat on the skin.)

❖ **Tea-tree** essential oil is an incredibly effective antiseptic: dab it on to wounds, cuts or spots to conquer local infection.

❖ **Valerian** is regarded as an effective alternative to prescription sleeping pills. Look for valerian-based sleep remedies.

Not just skin deep

Cosmetics companies can use terms like "natural" and "organic" much more freely than producers of food or medicine. Your skin absorbs much of what you put on it, so you need to be careful which products you use.

When it comes to cosmetics, "natural" is an incredibly confusing term. Just how natural is natural? The answer is, in many cases, not very natural at all. In several countries, only one percent of the ingredients have to be derived from nature for that word to be used. In fact, according to Dr. Jurgen Klein, founder of the Australian company Jurlique, one of the most natural skin care ranges available, "natural is the most abused term in the cosmetics industry today."

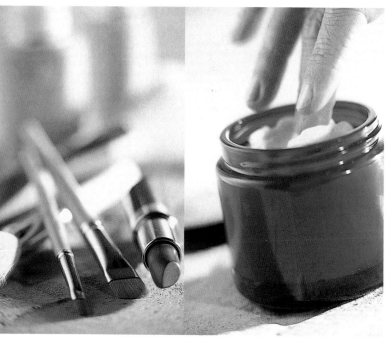

Now that organic food is popular, the word "organic" is also being hijacked by the conventional cosmetics industry. Since, as yet, the industry is not bound by the same sort of organic regulations as the food industry, it is hard for the shopper to tell what is really organic, and what may contain just a tiny amount of organic herbs, topped up with chemicals. However, a few companies are honest enough to list the percentage of organic ingredients in their products. The one product you may find carrying an organic symbol is toothpaste (*see page 138*), which can now be certified, in the UK, by the Soil Association if it meets their strict food criteria.

your skin is precious

There are important reasons for turning to "greener" cosmetics. It is easy to regard skin as just a covering for your body's organs, but in fact the skin itself is the body's largest organ. And in the last decade, the medical profession has done a huge turnaround. Not so long ago, they were telling us that the skin was a one-way street: sweat, oil, water, and toxins came out, but skin was basically as impermeable as a raincoat. Now all that has changed. Talk to doctors today and they describe skin as a "sponge" – which is why it is now being used as a delivery system for patches to wean smokers off cigarettes or to apply drugs like hormone replacement therapy. According to Charlotte Voght, founder of the British cosmetics brand the Green People's Company, women may absorb up to 4.4 lb (2 kg) of chemicals through their skin every year. Indeed, Rob McCaleb, president of the Herb Research Foundation in Boulder, Colorado, insists that "as much as 60 percent of any substance applied to the skin is absorbed into the body. So you should choose your cosmetics with as much care as the foods you eat."

In this section you can find easy steps that you can take right now to make the shift towards more organic, more natural skincare. And it is important to remember that your purse has a lot of power. In the same way that support for organic food companies has vastly widened the choice of what is available, encouraging more farmers to go organic as they see the market's potential, soaring sales of natural cosmetics will make beauty companies – maybe even the big ones – start to think about change, too. So it is worth buying organic beauty products when you see them.

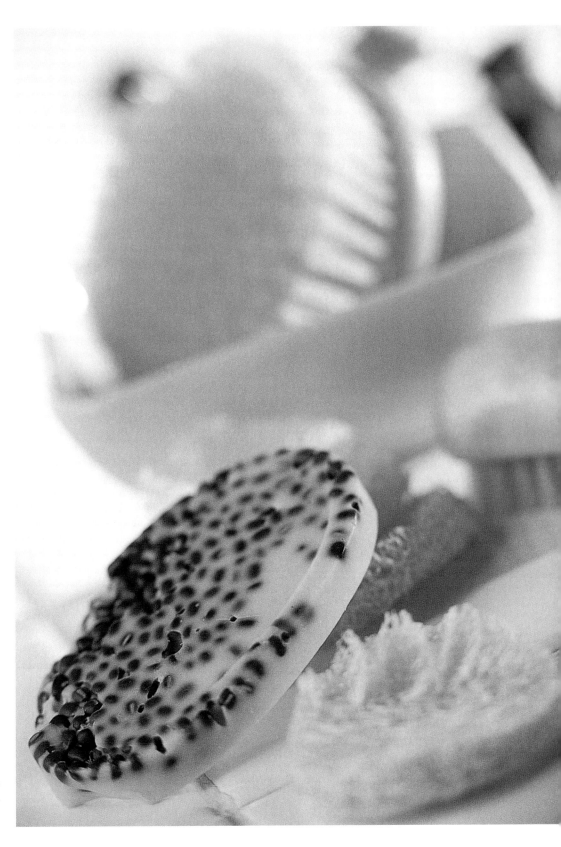

Not just skin deep

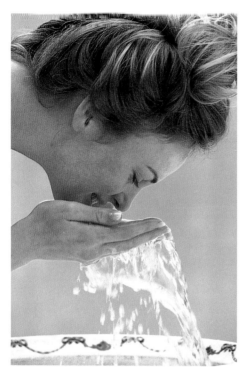

bodycare

When it comes to body care, for instance, the square footage of body skin means that you're potentially exposed to a much higher level of chemicals than, say, via your light nightly dab of eye cream. (The sheer speed with which you get through a bottle of body lotion should tell you that.) So, instead of creams, try moisturizing the body with oils such as jojoba, almond, or grapeseed, to which a few drops of essential oils have been added. That way,

you will avoid the long list of preservatives which go into many body creams and lotions, since many essential oils are naturally preservative. Nevertheless, keep bottles away from sunlight to maximize their shelf-life and prevent them becoming rancid.

lipstick

Another product to put high on your natural and organic shopping list is lipstick. According to the founder of the American natural cosmetics company Aveda, Horst Rechelbacher, lipstick-wearers consume anything from one-and-a-half to four tubes of lipstick in a lifetime. Companies making natural alternatives include Aveda, Jurlique, and Dr. Hauschka (*see right*).

avoiding petrochemicals

You happily put gas in your car. But did you realize that you are almost certainly putting it on your face and body, too? Propylene glycol, mineral oil, and petrolatum figure high on the ingredients list of most skin care, body care, and hair care products, and even many of the big-

name, so-called "natural products" are based on petrochemicals. Petroleum-derived ingredients are among the most common preservatives used in the cosmetics industry. Even though the amount that goes into a moisturizer is probably tiny compared to the fuel used to drive to the shop to buy it, by continuing our reliance on petrochemicals we head down a one-way street that ends with environmental disaster.

Globally, we should be increasing plant growth and decreasing pollution. Switching from fossil fuel derived ingredients to plant elements is an important and easy step in the process. They may be more expensive – naturally derived alternatives can cost up to 10 or 20 times more than petrochemical ingredients – but they are actually cheap if we consider the environmental cost. In reality, ingredient costs are usually only a small part of the final bill you pay for a beauty or personal-care product. Packaging, manufacturing costs, transportation, even tax all add a lot more to the price of any product. So look for products that say "free of petrochemicals" or "no petrochemical ingredients" on the label. You may pay a bit more – but think of it as an investment in our planet.

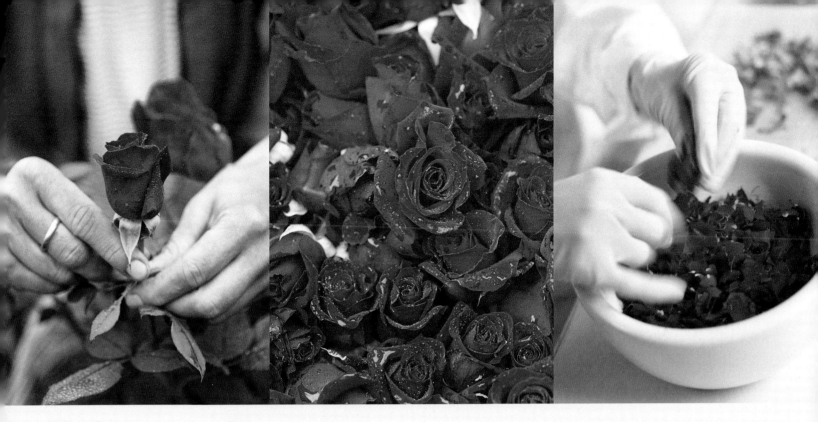

the producers

DR. HAUSCHKA

Organic beauty is nothing revolutionary for Dr. Hauschka, the German beauty manufacturer whose fans include Cher, Jerry Hall, and Jack Nicholson. It has been producing "holistic" cosmetics for more than 30 years, using the most exacting methods: harvesting flowers at dawn to capture their full "life force", ensuring that workers are in the right "calm and meditative" mood before making the products, and even cleaning bowls with feathers. There can be few other companies that put as much care and thought into a jar of face cream.

Dr. Hauschka himself was a chemist and creator of herbal remedies who was highly influenced by Dr. Rudolf Steiner – a pioneer of natural living who believed in creating a balance between the physical and spiritual worlds in every area of daily living, treating the mind and spirit as well as the body to ensure total well-being.

METHODS & INGREDIENTS

Ingredients come not only from the company's own fields and approved farms, but also from local hedgerows and woodlands. They are grown and harvested in line with the principles of biodynamic agriculture (*see page 43*), which takes organic growing one stage further. Traditionally, foresters cut wood at different times of the month, depending on what the wood was to be used for. For example, Stradivarius made sure the wood for his violins was cut only during certain phases of the moon; Dr. Hauschka applies the same philosophy to its skin creams. In the same way, a facial or other treatment from a Dr. Hauschka practitioner will be tailored not only to each individual but also to the time of day and the season.

In a world where cosmetics are, in some cases, created by ex-NASA scientists using 21st-century technology, Dr. Hauschka's back-to-nature approach proves that it is possible to create effective skin care – and, most recently, make-up – without resorting to the use of undesirable synthetic preservatives and chemicals.

A natural smile and more

If you are concerned about the products you use on your skin, you should be even more careful about those you choose for your teeth, nails, or scalp. The products you use can contain a range of synthetic chemicals.

As with skin care, body care products and make-up, it is still difficult to find all-natural – or even as-natural-as-possible – shampoos and toothpastes. But if you are choosing to go organic because you are concerned about your own health, and not just that of the planet, you may decide that it is even more important to seek out an organic toothpaste than a moisturizer or a mascara. The reason? Some parts of the body, including the gums and scalp, are more absorbent than others, making it easier for chemicals to pass into the bloodstream.

toothpaste

It is logical that a toothpaste should be the first nonfood product in the world to be given an organic symbol; after all, it goes in our mouths and some, inevitably, gets swallowed. In fact, if someone has gum disease, with gums that bleed, it is a real short-cut for the chemicals in toothpaste to get into the bloodstream. However, in the quest for whiter, brighter smiles, many toothpastes have gone the opposite, high-tech route by adding chemicals like fluoride. Although fluoride can help fight tooth decay, it has been linked to an increase in bone fractures, and natural health experts believe it interferes with the body's balance of calcium, magnesium, iron, and zinc.

Of course, life is full of compromises. We constantly have to make decisions about what matters to us, and change our shopping habits accordingly. You might choose to follow your dentist's advice to use a fluoride toothpaste – or instead, choose a natural toothpaste and take other positive steps to prevent cavities. These might include cutting out sugar, getting plenty of vitamins, flossing your teeth regularly, and eating calcium-rich foods like dried peas and beans, dark, leafy greens (including beet and turnip tops and kale), and canned fish.

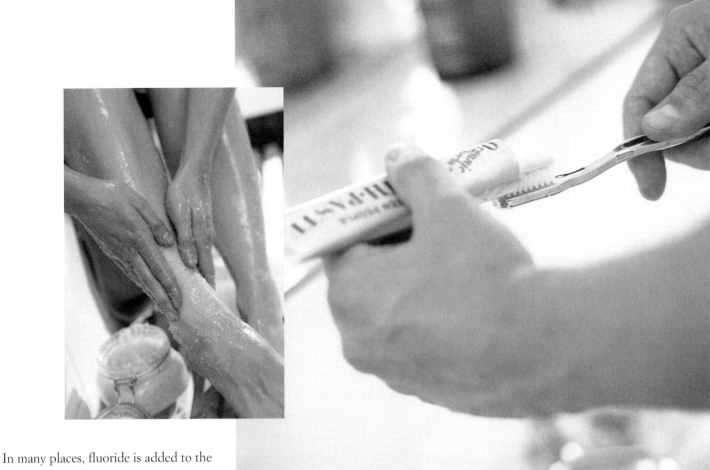

In many places, fluoride is added to the water supply – so you cannot avoid it simply by switching toothpastes. However, you can remove all traces of this chemical from the water that comes out of the tap by using a reverse osmosis water filter fitted in your kitchen.

nails

When it comes to nail products, hardeners, and polishes are, by definition, chemical-based. There is just no such thing as a natural nail polish, let alone an organic one. However, there are a couple of common ingredients which have been linked with allergies – in particular toluene and formaldehyde. You may not associate the use of nail polish with, for instance, itchy eyes or a face rash, but sensitivity to these ingredients is not restricted to the nail area, because we touch our faces so often. The good news is that it's getting easier all the time to find polishes which are free of toluene and formaldehyde, so seek these out.

If the reason you choose to wear polish is because your nails tend to flake and break, they can actually be strengthened over time by rubbing the same oil you use on your body into the cuticles and nail bed every night. As the nails grow out, they will be stronger and more flexible – in contrast to nails on which nail hardener has been used, which tend to become more brittle, snapping easily.

bath & shower

Instead of using detergent-based foams and gels, which can dry the skin, try switching instead to aromatherapy-based bath oils. These are products in which essential oils have been blended into "carrier" oils. Essential oils act as natural preservatives in these blends, so artificial chemical preservatives are unnecessary. Oils also replenish skin, leaving it silky. You can buy bath foams and gels blended in natural food stores, or learn to blend your own. Another natural option is bath salts infused with aromatherapy oils.

A natural and smile more

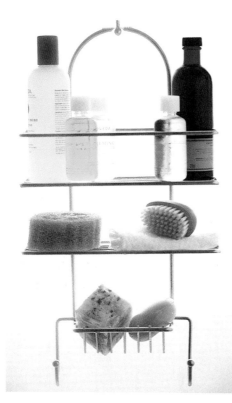

hair care

Shampoo is another personal care product where seeking out a natural alternative should be a shopping priority. The scalp – especially the pate of the head – is the most absorbent zone of the body, particularly when the skin is softened by washing, showering, and rinsing. If you cannot find ultra-natural shampoos and conditioners, the first step is to scan ingredients and avoid those with artificial fragrances and synthetic colors.

Do not be misled into thinking a shampoo is organic just because it contains a few organic herbs (as some recent launches by major international hair care companies do). These organic ingredients will, in reality, feature way down the ingredients list as a tiny percentage of the overall mix. While it is a step in the right direction for major haircare companies to source plant-based elements that have been more sustainably produced, a sprig of organic rosemary or mint does not make an organic shampoo.

TEN THINGS YOU DO NOT WANT IN YOUR NATURAL COSMETICS

❖ **Artificial colors** – several colors permitted in cosmetics are thought, by some experts, to be potential carcinogens. In particular, steer clear of the colors FD&C Red No. 6 and D&C Green No. 6. A natural-colored product does not mean it has no artificial colors, but avoiding rainbow shades should minimize your exposure to artificial dyes.

❖ **Formaldehyde** – an effective preservative used in nail hardeners, nail polish, and many cosmetics; however, skin reactions can be quite common, and some doctors worry about other more serious long-term effects.

❖ **Imidazolidinyl urea** – a widely used synthetic cosmetic preservative (and the second most commonly identified preservative causing contact dermatitis, according to the American Academy of Dermatology).

❖ **Fragrance** – the synthetic fragrances used in cosmetics may have as many as 200 ingredients, which do not have to be labeled separately. Some of the problems potentially caused by these chemicals are dizziness, rashes, hyperpigmentation, skin irritation, and more. However, "fragrance-free" is not a way of avoiding the problem, because smell-masking chemicals will usually have been added. Look for the words "natural fragrance" or choose products whose scent comes from essential oils.

❖ **Isopropyl alcohol** – an antibacterial solvent, derived from petroleum (which may also be used in anti-freeze).

❖ **Methyl paraben** – one of the most widely used preservatives. It may trigger irritation on sensitive skins (as can butyl, ethyl, and propyl paraben), and there is now some suggestion that these may all possibly be xenestrogens, or potential "gender bender" chemicals.

❖ **Methylisothiazolinone** – a preservative with a greater-than-normal potential for causing allergic reactions or irritation.

- **Paraffin** – used in cold creams, wax-based hair removers, eyebrow pencils, and a variety of other cosmetics. It is quite commonly derived from petroleum or coal.
- **Propylene glycol** – other than water, the most common moisture-carrying vehicle in cosmetics. Although it is possible to derive propylene glycol from vegetable glycerine, it is more usually derived from petroleum.
- **Sodium lauryl sulphate** – a commonly used detergent and emulsifier that may cause drying of the skin. This is because it has a degreasing effect, which can cause irritation.

There are alternatives to artificial chemical preservatives. Scan products' labels and look for these gentle and effective natural preservatives instead: grapefruit seed extract phenoxyethanol, potassium sorbate, sorbic acid, tocopherol (vitamin E), retinyl (vitamin A), and ascorbic acid (vitamin C).

the producers

AN INDIVIDUAL APPROACH

"We use soap every day – so why not try to make it in a way that is less harmful to the earth's resources?" says Nickki Clark of Woodspirits, who produces hand-made, almost-good-enough-to-eat soap in a South London warehouse. Since soap began to be mass-produced in the late 19th century, manufacturers have taken out its natural glycerine to make a harder bar that has a longer shelf life. "Handmade soap retains the glycerine, so it doesn't last as long – but it makes for a much gentler and more moisturizing bar," explains Nickki, whose soaps use food-grade olive and coconut oils, added therapeutic aromatherapy ingredients such as juniper and lavender, and natural colors such as ultramarine.

TRADITIONAL TECHNIQUES

"After you've worked with natural ingredients for a while, you begin to realize why manufacturers use chemicals. Producing a perfect bar every time is just not possible." Nevertheless, Nickki would not dream of changing the way she makes soap and trading her wooden paddle for high-tech machinery. "It's more like cooking than manufacturing," she explains.

Because everything is handmade, things can go wrong. However, scraps and failures are not wasted; they are chopped and re-mixed to make a multi-colored product called Salad Bar.

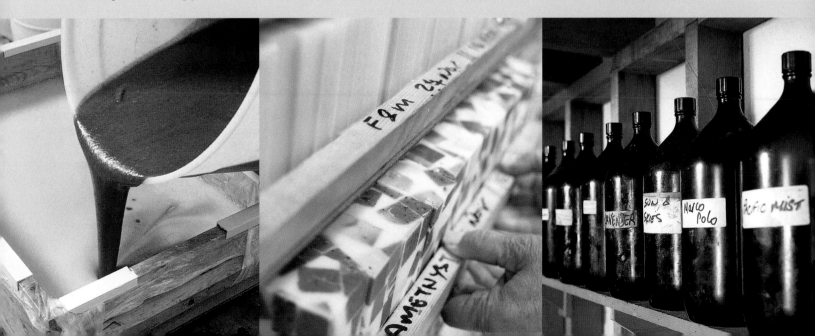

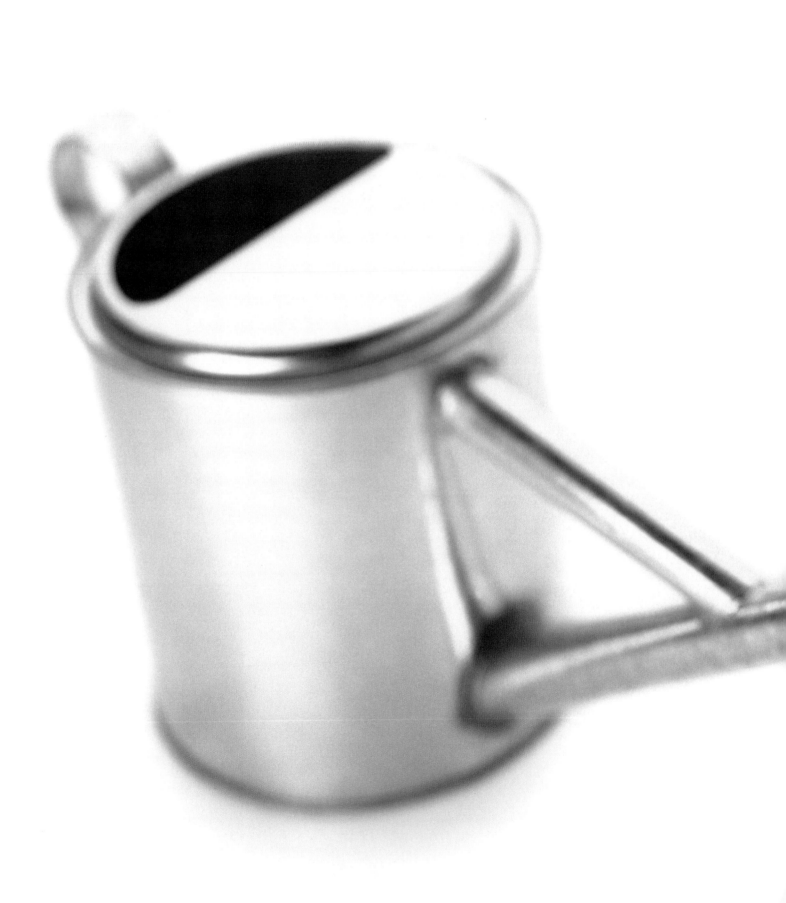

organic
GARDENING

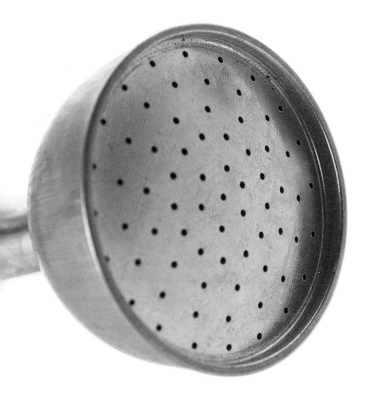

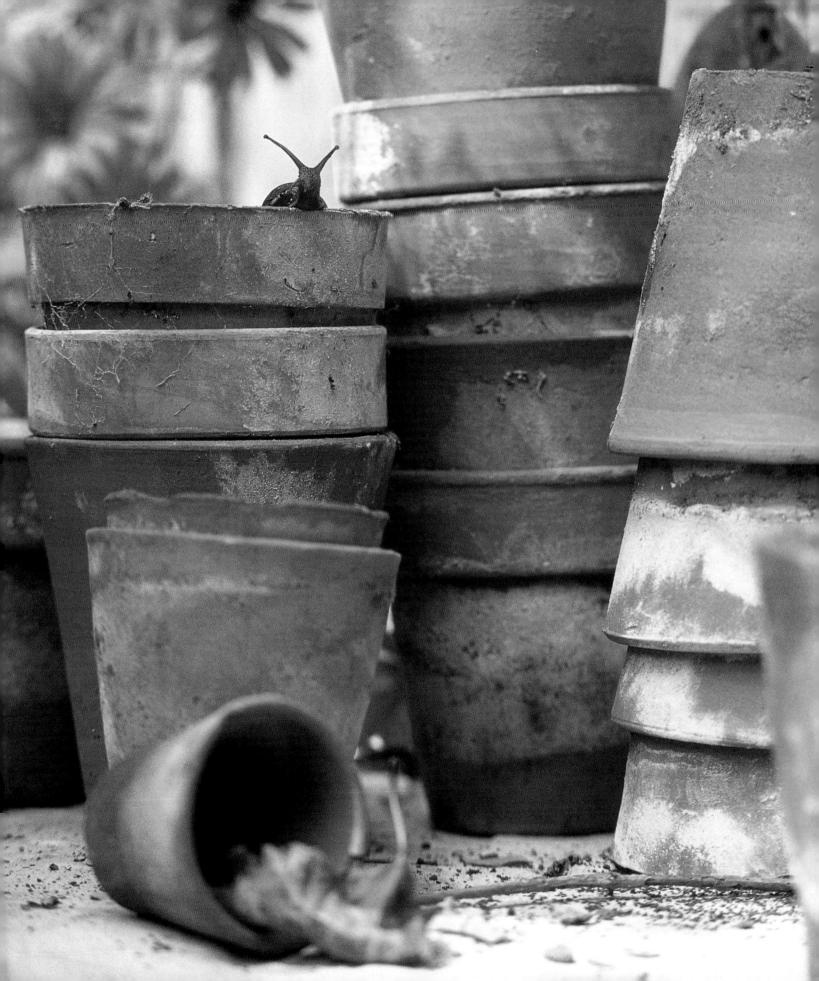

WHY GO organic

Organic gardens come in all shapes and sizes. They are packed with a wide variety of plants and reflect not just the diversity of nature, but also the diversity of the people who look after them.

Your garden is your own personal bit of paradise, where you are free to express yourself in any way you want. You might like to create your own floral wonderland or a productive plot for fresh fruit and vegetables. The priority could be a play area for the children or a relaxing haven in which to unwind after a hard day's work. Or you might want to do your bit for conservation: with natural areas rapidly dwindling in many areas, our yards and gardens can be valuable nature reserves, and organic methods support and attract wildlife. Whatever you want from your yard and garden areas, you can do it organically.

THE MEETING PLACE

A garden is where people and nature meet most directly. You only have to sit in any garden for a few minutes to notice some of the many creatures that call it home. And of course there are all the small-to-microscopic creatures which we tend to forget about – the ladybugs, for example, which

are eating aphids and other pests; the microscopic fungi and bacteria that are processing plant remains to recycle their goodness for growing plants; the bacteria vacuuming up nitrogen from the air to feed your garden. These creatures are all part of nature's plan – without them our gardens would not grow.

So, rather than a confrontation and collision, it is sensible to make that meeting with nature mutually beneficial, which is where organic gardening comes in. The basic idea of organic gardening is to harness and promote natural systems as far as possible, while also employing a wide range of other "nature-friendly" techniques to get what we want from the garden. If that all sounds much too complicated, take heart – it is not, as this chapter makes clear.

If you are new to organic gardening, why not join a local or national organic gardening group? Seeing is believing, too, so why not visit an organic garden open to the public for inspiration? Some of the resources listed in the back of this book will be happy to direct you to gardens near you.

Cultivate plants that support and attract wildlife

Choose eco-friendly products for your garden

Grow native or unusual varieties to help protect biodiversity

Visit an organic garden or two for inspiration

Join a local or national organic gardening group

What is organic gardening?

Organic gardening is an approach to gardening that emphasizes the importance of observing and cooperating with natural cycles, minimizing pollution, and promoting sustainability.

ORGANIC GARDENING

❖ Respects the environment

❖ Produces healthy food

❖ Encourages wildlife

❖ Recycles waste

❖ Reduces pollution

❖ Builds on traditional good gardening practice

❖ Embraces new technology where appropriate

❖ Makes use of local resources

There is no absolute definition of what organic gardening means, unlike commercial organic food production, which is regulated by enforceable standards (*see page 244*).

CONSUMER POWER – BUY ORGANIC

There is an increasing range of products available for the organic gardener to purchase, including soil mixes, manures, fertilizers, pest controls,

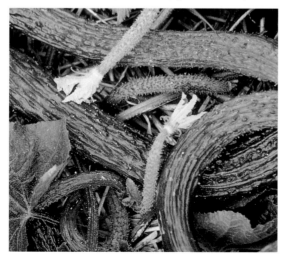

plants, seeds, and bulbs. It is not always easy to decide which particular brand or product to buy for an organic garden, as gardening products are not covered by the laws which regulate organic food certification and sale. The word "organic" can be used simply to mean "of living origin", and this may appear on fertilizers, manures, and similar items. Such products may, or may not, be suitable for use in an organic garden. Manure from a battery chicken farm, for example, could be labeled "organic" but, because it comes from an intensive farming system and is likely to contain unwanted pollutants, it would not be appropriate to use it in an organic garden. If in doubt, check with the supplier or manufacturer. Some brands do, however, carry a recognized organic symbol – which means that it has been certified by a registered organic body. Make them as your first choice. Seeds, bulbs, and plants that have an organic symbol will have been produced according to commercial organic

THE ORGANIC GARDENER'S SHOPPING BASKET

Select products that carry a recognized organic symbol where possible

Buy timber from sustainable sources, not tropical hardwoods that are nonsustainable

Choose products that are based on recycled and renewable ingredients

Use locally produced compost from green waste

Grow wildflower seeds of US origin

Avoid peat and products containing peat

Reject any animal manure products from intensive farming systems

Never buy bulbs taken from the wild or stone taken from ecologically sensitive areas

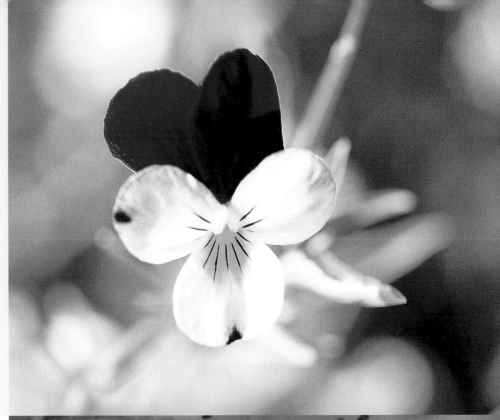

standards. Several seed companies are now able to supply organically grown seed, seed potatoes, and bulbs, and the range of varieties grows every year. Organic ornamentals and vegetable transplants are less commonly found. Keep asking, to let your usual supplier know that the demand is there and that your money will follow.

GARDEN HARDWARE

Gardening is not just about soil and plants – there is the fence, the garden furniture, the play-surface materials, and so on to consider, not forgetting the charcoal used in the barbecue. Again, there are no definitive standards covering this aspect of gardening as yet, although these will probably come as producers react to consumer demands. Where possible, exercise your purchasing power to buy products with low environmental impact, researching and considering the energy and pollution involved in production and distribution.

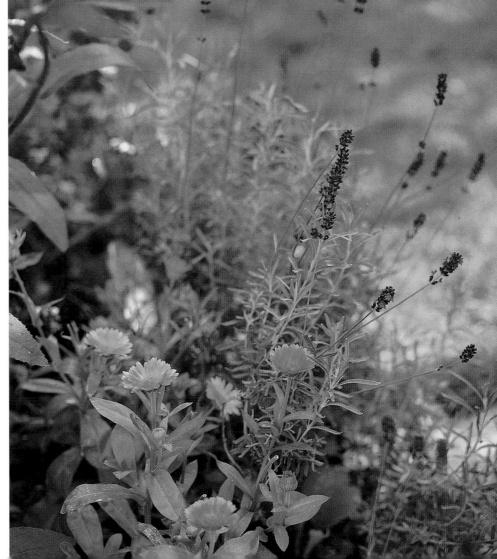

Plotting for success

Whether you are making changes to an existing garden, or starting afresh, it is worth spending a little bit of time on planning and preparation when you go organic.

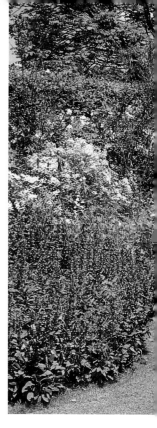

Grow your own organic fruit and vegetables at a fraction of the cost of store-bought ones

Create a safe play area for children and pets, free from pesticides and weed killers

Help the local environment by recycling garden and household waste: more than 50 percent could be composted or otherwise recycled in an organic garden

Produce pesticide-free flowers to cut for the house: many cut flowers sold are grown with heavy pesticide treatments

Help save a peat bog or a rainforest: organic gardeners avoid using peat or other materials whose production has had a negative impact on the environment

The best thing about organic gardening is that all of us can do it, no matter what our age, background or interests. The best way to start is to make a commitment to using organic methods throughout the whole garden. Use the checklist (*see far right*) to find out how organic you already are and to establish what simple steps you can take to improve the organic status of your garden.

The ideal organic garden will be attractive and easy to look after. It will also have the minimum possible negative impact on the environment. The best way to achieve this is by thoughtful and imaginative planning.

DESIRES & NECESSITIES

What you actually want from your garden will depend on your individual circumstances and personal taste. A busy professional is most likely to appreciate low-maintenance features, while for others priorities might include, for example, a place to contemplate wildlife, grow vegetables,

or accommodate a wading pool. Almost all of us need a hose, and all organic gardens, regardless of size or style, will definitely benefit from a compost pile.

Ask yourself what the most important elements are in a garden for you personally. Consider these carefully, be realistic about what can be achieved and do not hesitate to ask opinions of anyone who will share the garden.

ADAPT & SUCCEED

A successful organic garden will make the most of the natural features that already exist, developing these rather that trying to overcome them. A damp area might be an ideal spot for a bog garden, for instance, while salt-tolerant plants will flourish in a seaside garden and an infertile lawn would be a good place to develop a wildflower meadow. Careful observation of your garden will help you find out what plants will thrive in its particular conditions.

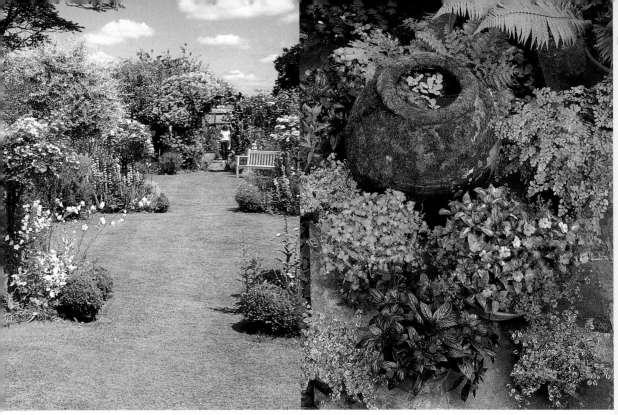

THE BEST LAID PLANS

Planning for success at the design stage can definitely help you avoid problems later on. Choose plants that suit your site to give them the best chance for healthy growth. Thorough preparation before planting or laying paths will help to prevent weeds emerging. Careful selection of plants and provision of habitats that attract wildlife will help boost your garden's natural defences (*see page 156*).

GARDEN WITH STYLE

Organic methods apply to all sorts of gardening styles, from a tiny city rooftop terrace to a vast natural wild flower meadow – and everything in between, too. The way you choose to garden depends to a large extent on how much time you actually want to devote to gardening, the energy and resources you have available, and what pleases you. Let your imagination run riot: there are no limits.

Baskets, tubs, and containers – these are excellent for a moveable display of flowers all year round, and are essential for a yard or patio. Some vegetables and herbs are also suitable for growing in different types of container. Be sure to provide adequate water and liquid feed during the growing season.

Climbers, trellises, and bowers – make use of the vertical nature of climbing plants to cover walls and fences, and to provide fragrant shade on garden structures. Try colorful gourds as an interesting alternative to flowering plants.

Herb spiral or wheel – organic herbs are a "must" for the kitchen. Growing them in a spiral shape shows off their ornamental value beautifully, or you could use the shape of a wheel to form a simple and effective design.

Raised beds – permanent structures can be raised to waist height. This not only brings plants within convenient reach, but also creates different levels in a garden. Lower, less elaborate beds are

Down to earth

The soil is a living organism that needs our respect and attention if it is to remain in top condition. Healthy soil rewards you with beautiful, vibrant plants and lies at the very heart of organic gardening.

COMMON ORGANISMS THAT LIVE IN THE SOIL

NAME	COMMENTS
Ants	help soil structure; some can sting; may encourage aphids
Bacteria and fungi	help soil structure; recycle nutrients; some types are harmful to plants
Beetles	eat pests
Centipedes	eat pests
Earthworms	help soil structure; recycle nutrients
Millipedes	eat some plant roots; recycle nutrients
Mites	recycle nutrients; eat pests; some can damage plants
Nematodes	some species can be pests; recycle nutrients
Slugs and snails	eat plants, but recycle nutrients
Spiders	eat pests

Healthy soil lies at the very foundations of good organic practice for both farmers and gardeners alike (*see page 16*). If it is properly nurtured, your soil will reward you with a garden teeming with life and strong, healthy plants.

ALIVE & WRIGGLING

As well as mineral particles of different sizes, soil contains water, plant roots, air, decaying organic matter, and living organisms. The organisms that live in the soil are very important in creating and maintaining its health (*see left*). Their job is to recycle plant and animal remains, breaking them down into forms that plants can make use of and absorb as nutrients.

A MATTER OF TIME

Soil texture refers to the different sizes of the mineral particles in the soil. There is nothing you as a gardener can do to alter the basic texture of your soil, which is formed by the weathering of

GARDENING WITH DIFFERENT TYPES OF SOIL

SOIL TYPE	CHARACTERISTICS	BENEFITS	DIFFICULTIES	CARE & MAINTENANCE
Mainly sandy soil	❖ often pale in color ❖ feels gritty between fingers ❖ will not form a ball when squeezed in the palm of the hand	❖ warms up fast in spring ❖ good for root crops and drought-tolerant plants ❖ easy to dig ❖ can be worked for most of the year ❖ drains easily	❖ dries out quickly ❖ nutrients are washed out easily	❖ add plenty of organic matter ❖ grow green manures ❖ do not leave bare in winter ❖ use minimum cultivation ❖ avoid heavy irrigation
Mainly clay soil	❖ sticks to tools and boots when wet ❖ feels sticky between fingers ❖ forms a ball easily when squeezed in the palm of the hand ❖ sometimes gray or yellow	❖ can be very fertile ❖ can grow a wide range of plants if well-structured	❖ drains slowly and may become waterlogged ❖ forms deep cracks when very dry ❖ difficult to dig ❖ warms up slowly in spring	❖ add plenty of organic matter ❖ grow green manures ❖ do not cultivate when wet ❖ avoid walking on when wet

rocks over thousands of years. Sand and clay are the two extremes of soil texture and most soils contain a mixture of these in varying proportions.

WHAT TYPE ARE YOU?

The type of soil you have will determine which sort of plants will grow best in it and how you need to look after it. To find out which you have in your garden, dig up a handful of soil. If dry, add just enough water to make it hold together. Rub it between your fingers, examine it carefully, and then compare it to the chart (*see above*).

THE JAM JAR TEST

Another test you can do to find out more about the soil in your garden involves filling a jar about two-thirds full with soil. Add enough water to fill the jar to the top and then secure the lid firmly.

Shake thoroughly, then let the contents to settle. Do not be surprised if this takes a day or so. The soil will settle into layers, with the largest particles (sand) at the bottom and the smallest (clay) on the top. Any bits floating on the surface will be organic matter. This simple test gives you a rough idea of the different proportion of particles in your soil.

STRUCTURALLY SOUND

The way that mineral particles are combined with other components in the soil is known as structure. Good soil structure is essential because it enables you to get the best possible results from your soil, whatever soil type you have. Unlike soil texture, structure is definitely something that can be affected by the way you treat it – for better or worse.

TYPICAL SIGNS OF POOR SOIL STRUCTURE

❖ Few earthworms present
❖ Plant roots do not penetrate deeply
❖ Compacted ground
❖ Poor plant growth
❖ Soil hard or dusty when dry
❖ Soil sticky and dense when wet
❖ Moss may grow on surface of soil

Organic gardening feeds your soul as well as your plants.

JACKIE GEAR, EXECUTIVE DIRECTOR, HDRA – THE ORGANIC ORGANIZATION

Down to earth

THE BENEFITS OF A COMPOST PILE

✤ It improves soil structure

✤ It provides long-term nutrients in a stable form

✤ It helps protect plants against diseases

✤ It reduces the need for bonfires

✤ It is free and saves money on bought products

✤ It keeps waste away from landfill sites

✤ It protects natural resources because it can be used instead of peat

CREATING A COMPOST PILE

Compost is a valuable and essential resource for the organic garden. It is the best tonic your garden can have, and it is free if you make your own.

There are many ways you can make your own compost. One of the quickest is to gather a lot of suitable material (*see chart opposite*) and construct a pile all at once. Many gardeners, however, find it more convenient to add material to their compost pile a little at a time, as and when it becomes available (*see far right*). This method produces good compost, although it may take 12–18 months, depending on the weather, to generate anything usable for the garden.

CHOOSING A CONTAINER

There are many different types of compost containers available to buy or make. Here are some points to consider when making your choice:

Weight – too light and it may blow over; too heavy and it becomes hard to move.

Cover – essential to keep moisture and warmth in, but to ensure rain stays out.

Base – one that is open to the ground for drainage is easiest to manage.

Appearance – choose something that suits the style of your garden.

Location – easy access is important, with enough space to maneuvre.

USING COMPOST

Your compost is ready to use when all trace of the original ingredients has disappeared and it is dark and crumbly with a sweet, earthy smell. There may also be some small red worms present, which help to produce a finely textured material. Use compost on those areas where you are going to grow plants that require a high level of nutrients. It is best applied to the soil in spring rather than autumn; otherwise, winter rain might wash out the nutrients. As a general guide, normal application rates are one barrowful to roughly 18 sq ft (5 sq m) of soil, repeated annually.

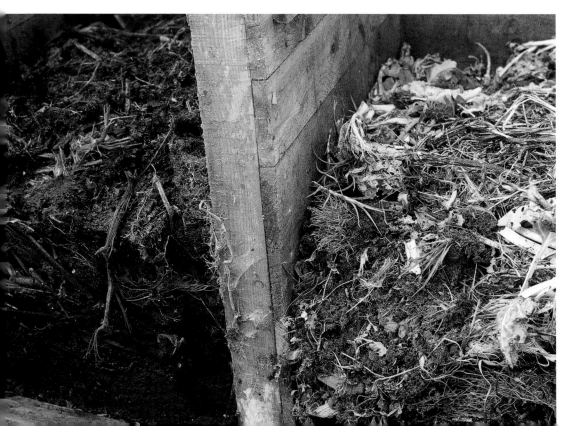

WHAT CAN YOU PUT ON YOUR COMPOST PILE?

Anything that has once lived will decompose, but this does not necessarily make it suitable for inclusion in a compost pile. Do not put synthetic materials on your compost pile, since they do not break down. Success depends on balancing soft, sappy materials with tougher, more fibrous ones.

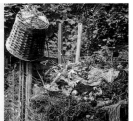

MATERIAL	BREAKS DOWN QUICKLY	BREAKS DOWN SLOWLY	DO NOT USE	COMMENTS
Cat litter or dog feces			●	can carry disease
Chicken manure	●			high in nutrients
Diseased plant material			●	some diseases may persist
Farmyard manure		●		add water if very dry
Grass clippings	●			mix well with dry materials
Household cardboard (egg boxes, cereal packages)		●		crumple and mix with wet materials, kitchen waste, or grass clippings
Kitchen scraps	●			mix with dry material
Mature garden waste		●		chop to aid breakdown
Meat or fish scraps			●	may attract pests
Newspaper		●		better to recycle in other ways; use small amounts, torn or shredded
Perennial weeds			●	may continue growing
Plastic, tin, glass			●	will not break down; can cause injury
Soft prunings		●		chop to aid breakdown
Large, woody prunings			●	too tough, will not break down fast enough
Young garden weeds	●			add before seeds form

SLOWLY DOES IT

Many gardeners make their compost using this method, which is slow but sure:

Gather a good mixture of materials to make layers roughly 12 in (30 cm) deep at a time.

Add materials to the pile, spread them out evenly and firm them down very gently or not at all.

Add water if the materials are very dry, then cover. Continue to add materials a bit at a time, balancing soft and tough ingredients.

Check and adjust moisture levels as necessary. Excess moisture makes the pile sludgy and smelly; too little slows decomposition.

The oldest material at the bottom of the pile will be ready first. If using a bin or a box, lift off the lid or remove the front as appropriate. Then separate the top and bottom layers retaining the mature bottom layer, which should be dark and crumbly. Return the rest to the pile, ready to start adding new material on top.

Speed up the process by turning the pile frequently, adding new material regularly, and using garden soil or compost starter to add the organisms that decompose the materials.

The quality of the food you eat comes from the quality of the soil it is grown in.

W. E. SHEWELL-COOPER, MBE, *SOIL, HUMUS AND HEALTH*, 1975

Down
to earth

INTRODUCING GREEN MANURES

You can actually grow plants that enrich and protect your soil (*see chart right*). Known as green manures, there are many types, suitable for different seasons and situations. Green manures help to protect the soil from wind and rain. They reduce weeds and, when incorporated into the soil, provide valuable organic matter and plant nutrients.

GROW YOUR OWN GREEN MANURE

Green manures can be grown throughout the year. You can grow them on bare areas of soil during the winter. In summer, cultivate them between different crops of vegetables. Growing them improves the fertility of your soil and prevents weeds taking over on any land you have that is not being used.

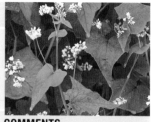

NAME	PREFERRED SOIL TYPE	SOWING TIME	WINTER HARDY	COMMENTS
Buckwheat (*Fagopyrum esculentum*)	tolerates poor soils	March – August	no	❖ deep-rooted ❖ flowers attract hoverflies
Crimson clover (*Trifolium incarnatum*)	dislikes heavy soil	March – August	sometimes	❖ large red flowers attract bees ❖ vigorous growth habit
Essex red clover (*Trifolium pratense*)	prefers good loam	April – August	yes	❖ deep-rooting, bushy plants ❖ flowers attract bees
Grazing rye (*Secale cereale*)	tolerates most types	August – October	yes	❖ extensive root system ❖ good weed control ❖ best dug in when young ❖ do not use before sowing fine seed (it inhibits germination)
Mustard (*Sinapis alba*)	needs moist soil	March – September	no	❖ very quick-growing ❖ susceptible to clubroot
Phacelia (*Phacelia tanacetifolia*)	tolerates most types	March – September	sometimes	❖ bright lavender/blue flowers attract bees and hoverflies ❖ good weed control
Winter field beans (*Vicia faba*)	likes heavy soil	September – November	yes	❖ not drought-tolerant ❖ poor weed control
Winter tares (*Vicia sativa*)	likes slightly heavy soil	March – May and July – September	yes	❖ rapid growth habit ❖ will not thrive on dry or acid soil

WHAT ELSE WORKS?

Other recycled materials you can use to improve your soil include:

Local compost – contact your local authority, as many operate programs that compost their green waste to produce a useful soil conditioner.

Autumn leaves – gather leaves to make leafmold, either stacking them in a wire-mesh container or stuffing them into heavy paper sacks for roughly 12 months (making sure the leaves stay moist). Spread the resulting leafmold freely on your soil to improve its structure.

Grass clippings – use as a mulch around your plants to control the weeds and improve the soil structure. You can leave your clippings on the lawn to recycle their nutrients.

Perennial weeds – Gather them up and store them in an isolated pile, keeping the weeds wet. When they have completely rotted, add them to the compost pile to take advantage of their valuable nutrients.

FEEDING TIME

A healthy soil that has regular applications of compost or other bulky material will normally be able to supply all the nutrients your plants need. However, you may sometimes find it necessary to provide extra nutrients in the form of fertilizers. This may be just because you do not have enough compost available, or it may be necessary due to the particular demands of a plant or to correct major deficiencies in the soil.

Fertilizers suitable for use in an organic garden are normally broken down gradually by the natural processes of decomposition, rather than providing the "quick fix" of available nutrients that most other fertilizers offer. When buying fertilizer products, be sure to look out for those

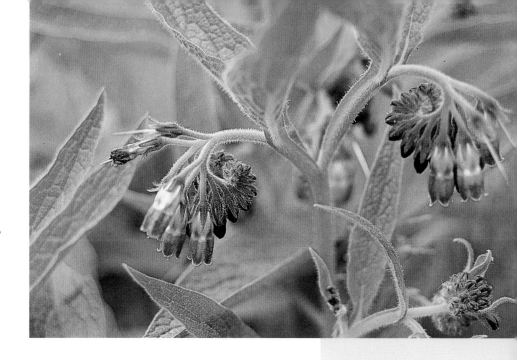

with organic certification (*see page 244*). Organic fertilizers can be derived from animal, plant, or mineral origin, such as the common types listed here:

Animal-based fertilizers – pelletted chicken manure, fish, blood, and bone meal, hoof and horn meal, wool or sheep waste, worm compost

Plant-based fertilizers – hop waste, vinash (a by-product of the sugar beet industry), seaweed meal, other recycled products

Mineral-based fertilizers – rock phosphate, limestone

FLUIDS THAT FERTILIZE

In organic gardens, liquid feeds are usually only used for plants growing in containers. Liquid feeds include liquid manure, fish emulsion, and comfrey liquid (*see above right*). Use them diluted as a foliar spray or apply them directly to the soil.

You can also use seaweed extract as a liquid tonic, although it does not contain enough major nutrients to be a fertilizer. It does have a good range of minor nutrients, though, so is excellent as a plant tonic and growth stimulant. Use it as a foliar spray to give plants a boost.

MAKING YOUR OWN COMFREY LIQUID

Comfrey (*see above*) is easy to grow, but needs quite a bit of space, so is not suitable for tiny gardens. Comfrey liquid is an excellent fertilizer for plants with flowers or fruit. But be warned – it is also very smelly.

METHOD

Cut some comfrey leaves and stuff them into a nylon net bag or leave them loose

Place the leaves in a large bucket, trashcan or barrel with a tight-fitting lid

Cover the leaves with water and put the lid on the container

Let to soak for four to six weeks

Strain off the liquid for use – it should be about the color of weak tea; if it is much darker, dilute it with water

Defense
of the domain

All gardeners want to keep their gardens healthy and as free of pests and diseases as possible. Organic gardeners, however, do not resort to harsh pesticides, preferring to work with nature rather than against it.

The organic approach to pests and diseases is to copy the way nature deals with them, as well as using other strategies to promote healthy plants. Organic gardeners let nature assist them in the defence of their gardens, encouraging natural predators such as birds, who can help keep the insect pest population at bay, and using labor-saving tricks such as mulching to control weeds and protect the soil.

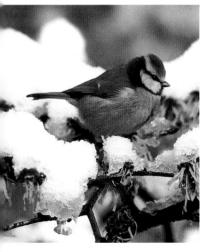

BEAT THE WEEDS
In an organic garden the aim is to control those weeds that threaten to overwhelm your plants, not to eliminate every one from the garden. Any plant can become a weed if it is growing in the wrong place or starts to take over. Different types of weeds need different measures (*see chart right*). Annual weeds have shallow roots, so you can easily hoe or dig them out by hand, but they may also produce carpets of seedlings. Perennial weeds have deep or creeping roots that are harder to dig

out. Unfortunately, just removing the top growth from these will not stop them regrowing. There are no chemical weed killers suitable for use in an organic system, so controlling the weeds in your garden relies on forking out, mulching, hand-weeding, hoeing, and cultivation. You may also find a flame weeder useful on hard surfaces and to kill seedlings.

MULCHING FOR WEED CONTROL
A mulch helps you control weeds by excluding light and therefore preventing plant growth. Some mulches are biodegradable, giving them the added benefit of improving the soil as they break down. These loose mulches need to be about 4–6 in (10–15 cm) deep. You can choose various types of mulch to create different effects, including gravel chippings, bark chips, and straw.

Mulching fabrics can be particularly effective. You can use newspaper or cardboard, or buy materials such as flax matting. These allow water

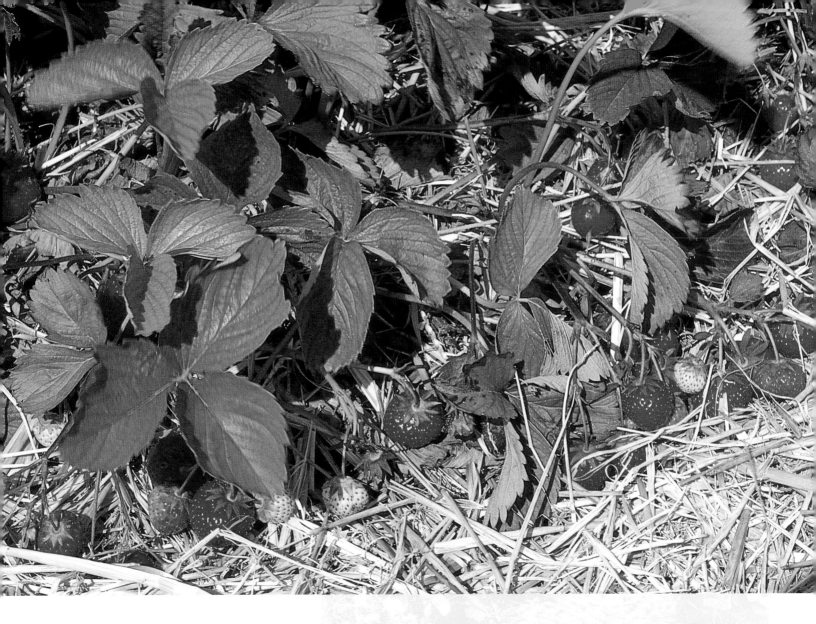

and air through while keeping weeds down. Mulch fabrics are usually covered with a thin layer of loose mulch to keep them in place, prolong their life, and improve their appearance.

CLEARING THE WAY
Digging the weeds in is a quick method of clearing ground that is practical for small areas, as long as all the roots of perennial weeds are removed. On larger areas you might prefer laying a mulch on top of the weeds instead. Heavy-duty black plastic and thick cardboard topped with leaves and straw are both suitable, or you can buy mulching fabrics. Leave

COMMON TYPES OF WEED CONTROL

WEED PROBLEM AREA	HOW TO MINIMIZE	HOW TO CONTROL
Flower and vegetable beds	control weeds when small; do not allow seeding	hand-weeding; hoeing; mulches
Paths and hard surfaces	thorough preparation before laying	hand-weeding; flame weeder; kitchen knife for crevices
Permanent planting	thorough preparation before planting; plant through a permeable membrane	hand-weeding for deep roots; hoeing for surface weeds; mulches
Trees, shrubs, and fruit bushes	thorough preparation before planting	hand-weeding; hoeing; mulches

Defense
of the domain

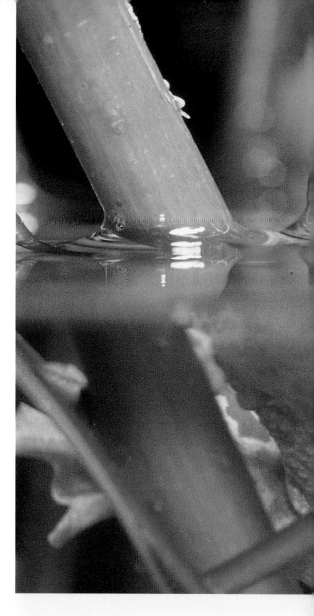

the mulch in place from spring to autumn to kill annual weeds and give perennial weeds a real setback. Any that remain can be dug out by hand, or you can keep the mulch in place for another six months or so. Top off biodegradable mulches as they decay. Remove black plastic after six months; replace it if necessary after a month or so, to allow the soil to breathe and rain to soak it.

PESTICIDE-FREE PEST CONTROL

There are plenty of steps you can take to limit the populations of common pests in your garden while still avoiding the use of artificial pesticides. Encouraging the natural enemies of pests (*see right*) can help, for example, so do your best to attract these beneficial creatures into your garden. Adjusting growing conditions, meanwhile, can help to limit the spread of diseases in your garden. In addition, there is a range of defensive measures you can take to protect your plants. By using a combination of these methods, it is possible to have a healthy garden without resorting to pesticides.

Small amounts of pests and diseases will not affect the health of your plants too seriously. If they get out of control, don't panic – there are some natural pest controls that can be used to help save a plant (*see page 162*). All plants do better in some gardens than others, so if a particular pest or disease is a problem in your area, try something different instead.

KNOW YOUR FRIENDS

Learn to recognize your natural allies and encourage them into your garden. Most of them will benefit from a garden that is not too neat and tidy, but you do not need to create a jungle. Shelter can be provided among undergrowth, tussocky grass, and hollow stems of herbaceous plants. Insects can be enticed into the garden by growing particular flowers (*see page 160*). Many beneficial creatures are very sensitive to toxic chemicals, so avoid using sprays or poisons of any kind.

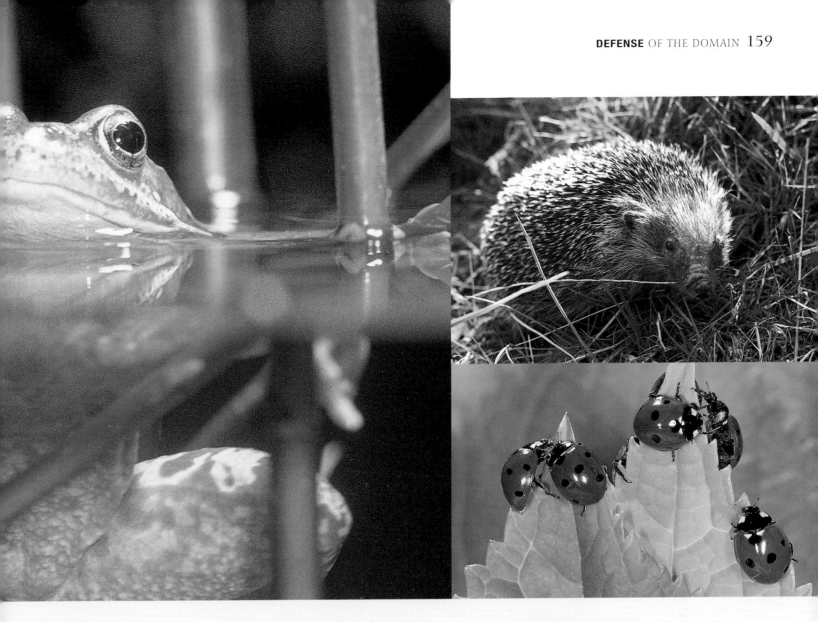

BATS
❖ eat insect pests

❖ attract them by growing plants that attract insects and by putting up bat boxes

BIRDS
❖ eat insects pests on plants and in the soil

❖ attract them by providing food, water, and shelter: some can damage plants, but it is still worth encouraging them into the garden, protecting susceptible plants with nets or other methods

CENTIPEDES
❖ the adults eat soil-living and insect pests

❖ attract them by keeping your soil covered with mulches and providing bricks or tiles for shelter

FROGS & TOADS
❖ eat slugs; toads also eat snails and woodlice

❖ attract them by building a pond and providing damp, secure places for shelter

GROUND & ROVE BEETLES
❖ the adults and larvae eat slugs and other soil-living pests

❖ attract them by keeping your soil covered with mulches and providing bricks or tiles for shelter

HOVERFLIES
❖ the larvae eat aphids

❖ attract them by growing particular flowers to feed the adults

LACEWINGS
❖ the larvae eat aphids, caterpillars, scale insects and other pests

❖ attract them by growing particular flowers to feed the adults and providing shelter for hibernation

LADYBUGS
❖ eat aphids such as greenfly and blackfly

❖ attract them by growing a patch of nettles in a corner of your garden and providing shelter for hibernation

Defense
of the domain

BE ATTRACTIVE

Mix these attractive plants in among all the flowers, shrubs, and vegetables throughout your garden. Not only will they be appreciated for their appearance, but their simple, open flowers will provide easy access to pollen and nectar for beneficial insects.

✤ Annual convolvulus
(Convolvulus tricolor)

✤ Baby blue-eyes
(Nemophila insignis)

✤ California poppy
(Eschscholzia californica)

✤ Corn chamomile
(Anthemis arvensis)

✤ Cornflower
(Centaurea cyanus)

✤ Corn marigold
(Chrysanthemum segetum)

✤ Fennel
(Foeniculum vulgare)

✤ Poached egg plant
(Limnanthes douglasii)

✤ Pot marigold
(Calendula officinalis)

✤ Yarrow
(Achillea millefolium)

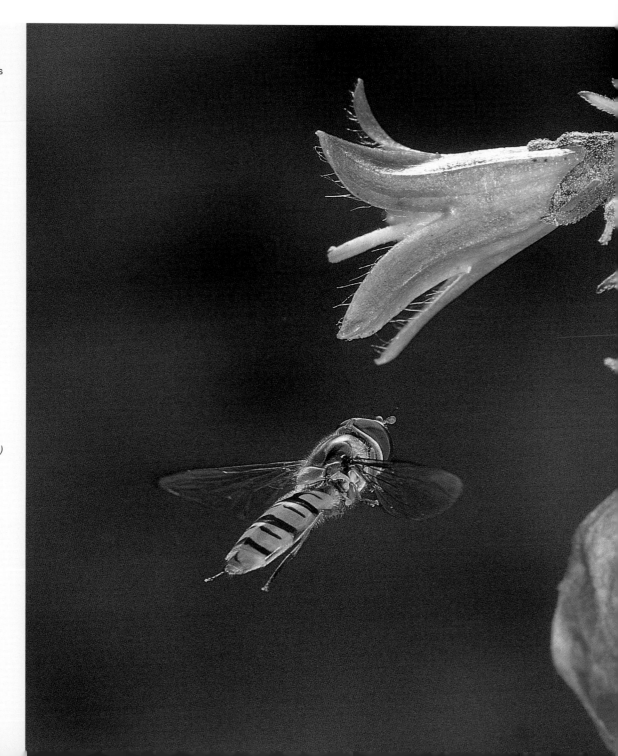

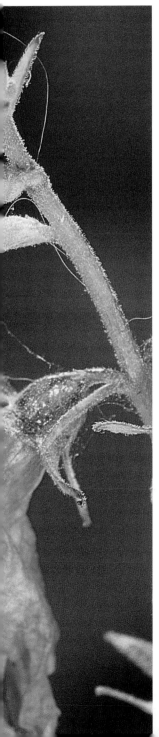

PREEMPTIVE STRATEGIES

Prevention is definitely the best form of defense when it comes to your garden. Aim to prevent problems from arising in the first place, and develop long-term strategies that will promote plant health throughout the whole garden. Make sure you look after your soil, since it is the starting place for healthy plant growth. Healthy plants are in a better position to withstand and recover from attack by pests and disease than weaker specimens.

Give them a good start – make sure your seedlings and transplants have the best growing conditions at all times. Never let them outgrow their pots or cell packs. When buying plants, avoid weak, straggly, or root-bound ones.

Maintenance – once established, make sure plants don't run short of nutrients or moisture by improving the soil and using mulches.

Do not crowd them – provide enough space for plants to grow to their full potential; overcrowding means competition for light, water, and nutrients, and makes it easier for pests or diseases to spread.

Location is everything – choose plants that will match the conditions you can provide. Acid-loving plants will struggle if the soil is too alkaline, for instance, while sun-loving plants will not thrive in a dark, damp corner.

Put on a variety show – a garden full of different plants all growing together is closer to a natural environment than regimented rows of the same thing. This makes it easier for the beneficial and harmful creatures to maintain a natural balance between each other. Mixed planting also looks attractive, giving a relaxed, informal feel to a garden.

Cut out the rot – carefully remove diseased material as soon as you spot it, to prevent it spreading. Do not add seriously diseased material to your compost pile.

Keep your eyes open – regularly inspect your plants and you are more likely to prevent problems getting out of control. Infection or infestation is more easily dealt with in the early stages. Removing pests by hand in the early stages is an efficient control method.

Build up your defenses – use protection such as fences, nets, and cloches to prevent pest damage. Crop covers such as horticultural fleece or mesh are useful against insects; set traps for slugs, earwigs, and sowbugs; and use scaring devices to deter birds, moles, and cats.

Organic gardening is often a cheaper, more economical way to garden and it's so much more satisfying: a way to get close to nature.

THELMA BARLOW, *ORGANIC GARDENING WITH LOVE*, 1992

Defense
of the domain

Choose resistant varieties – some varieties are naturally less susceptible to certain pests or diseases, and some have been specially developed to enhance these qualities. Check with your suppliers for resistant varieties of flowers, fruit, and vegetables.
Ring the changes – do not grow vegetables from the same family in the same place year after year

since this can encourage the buildup of pests and diseases. The same principle applies when replacing roses and fruit trees or bushes.
Timed to perfection – choose your sowing time carefully to avoid the periods when some pests and diseases are most active. Carrot rust fly and pea moth are two pests that can be controlled by sowing either early or late to avoid the main egg-laying periods.

BIOLOGICAL CONTROLS

Biological controls can be bought to help with pest control. These are living creatures that are available commercially. They are harmless to humans, pets, and beneficial creatures. Some are suitable only for use in your greenhouse or conservatory, while others can also be used outside. They are most effective if used at the earliest stages of infestation and are very sensitive to any sprays, even the ones described in our chart (*see left*). Biological controls are mostly available by mail order and need to be used immediately on, or soon after, delivery.

THE LAST RESORT

The sprays suitable for an organic system are generally of plant origin and biodegrade quickly. They are not completely harmless to beneficial creatures, so use them only as a last resort and do not rely on sprays alone to keep plants healthy.

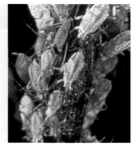

PRODUCT	TYPE	USE AGAINST	CAUTION
Rotenone	plant-based liquid or powder	aphids; sawfly; spider mites; thrips	poisonous to fish, ladybugs, other beneficial insects
Insecticidal soap	liquid based on fatty acids	aphids; spider mites; whitefly, and other insects	harmful to ladybugs and may damage some plants
Plant oil	liquid based on canola oil	aphids; scale insect; spider mite; thrips; whitefly	do not use on young plants, begonias, and fuchsias
Pyrethrum	plant-based liquid or powder	aphids; flea beetles; small caterpillars	poisonous to fish and beneficial insects
Sulphur	powder or liquid	powdery mildew; scab on fruit	causes damage to some plants; harmful to beneficial insects

SPRAYING DOS & DON'TS

❖ Do identify precisely what the problem is

❖ Do select the appropriate treatment (*see charts*)

❖ Do follow the manufacturer's instructions and use only as directed on the label

❖ Do spray in calm weather to avoid spray drift

❖ Do not spray where bees are present; wait until dusk when the bees are less active

SOME COMMON PROBLEMS — HOW TO PREVENT AND CONTROL THEM

PEST	PREVENTION	CONTROL
Aphids	attract natural enemies such as spiders; use protective covers	biological control (*Aphidoletes aphidimiza*), indoors only; insecticidal soap; rotenone; plant oil
Birds	use protective covers and scaring devices	none
Caterpillars	attract natural enemies such as birds and spiders; use protective covers; remove by hand	biological control (*Bacillus thuringiensis*), inside and out
Greenhouse spider mite	keep the atmosphere humid	biological control (*Phytoseiulus persimilis*), inside and out; pyrethrum
Greenhouse whitefly	sticky traps	biological control (*Encarsia formosa*), inside only; insecticidal soap
Rabbits	use fences, protective covers, and repellents	trapping
Slugs	attract natural enemies such as frogs and skunks; use protective covers, traps, or deterrents	biological control (*Phasmarhabditis hermaphrodita*), inside and out
Vine weevil	put nondrying glue around pots	check roots of plants for larvae, remove and destroy if found; collect and destroy adults; biological control (*Heterorhabditis megidis*), inside and out

DISEASE	PREVENTION	CONTROL
Blackspot on roses	grow resistant varieties; remove all fallen leaves in autumn; prune hard in spring and mulch	sulphur
Clubroot	improve drainage; make soil alkaline; use long rotation; do not compost infected plants	none
Potato blight	choose resistant varieties	remove affected foliage; do not harvest tubers for at least three weeks after foliage is removed
Powdery mildew	grow resistant varieties; encourage good air flow; remove sources of infection	sulphur
Rust	grow resistant varieties; collect and discard affected leaves in autumn	none
Virus	grow resistant varieties; destroy infected material; control aphids that spread the virus	none
White rot	dig out infected plants; do not add to compost pile	none

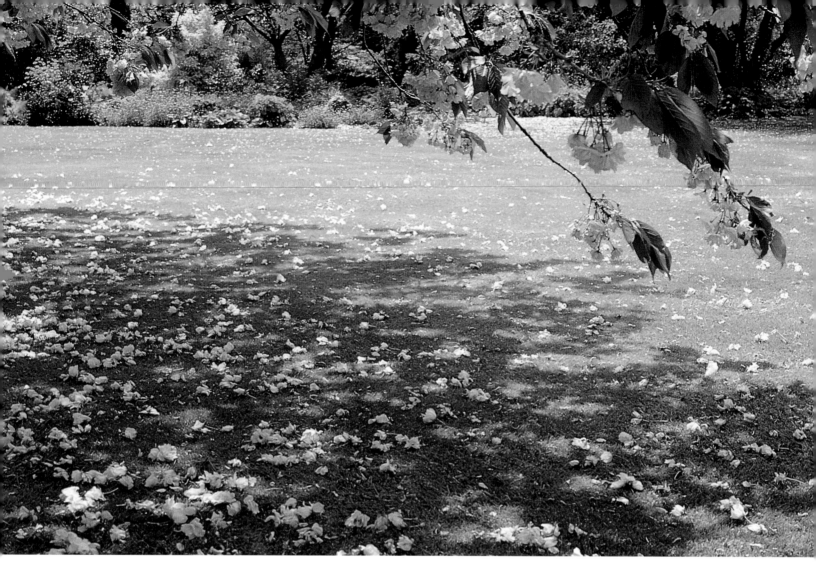

Magic carpets

There is nothing quite like strolling barefoot across a beautiful lawn and feeling the grass between your toes – especially if it is organic. A healthy organic lawn goes one step further.

Organic gardening is all about gardening for the future of the earth. One individual with a digging fork and a small garden can make a real difference.

HOWARD-YANA SHAPIRO PhD, AGRICULTURAL AND COMMERCIAL DIRECTOR, SEEDS OF CHANGE

A lush organic lawn is a beautiful feature in a garden of any size. If you want to keep your organic lawn in top condition, your best bet is to encourage the grass to grow well. This may involve a little bit of effort sometimes, such as raking hard in autumn to help remove dead material from the surface or spiking any compacted ground with a fork or mechanical aerator to loosen it up, but the results will be worth the time and energy expended. No matter how dry the weather, you can save yourself time and resources by not watering your lawn. Resist the urge – even if it starts looking brown, it will certainly recover once rain arrives.

OFF TO MOW

Your choice of lawnmower will depend on the size and condition of your lawn. An old-fashioned push-mower will produce the least pollution and, as an added bonus, provide you with maximum exercise. While suitable for a small lawn, however, this type of push-mower is not practical for long grass or rough, uneven areas, even if you are particularly energetic.

Cutting too severely will weaken your grass, allowing weeds to flourish. For a general-purpose lawn, you should aim to cut the grass to about 1¼ in (3 cm) in height. Contrary to popular opinion, the clippings can usually be left to lie on the lawn to provide nutrients as they break down. The exception is when the weather is cold and damp, or when the clippings are very long. In such cases you should add the clippings to the compost pile or use them as a mulch instead.

How often you need to get the lawnmower out depends on the season and weather. Cut your lawn when the grass reaches about 1¾ in (4.5 cm) in height, rather than sticking to a rigid timetable.

THE NEED TO WEED

Relax – there is no harm in allowing a few weeds within your lawn. If it is well managed, most of the weeds will be crowded out by strongly growing grass anyway.

Flat, spreading weeds such as plantain and dandelion should be dug out with a strong knife, making sure to remove as much of the roots as possible. If you have moss growing in your organic lawn, it is an indicator that the growing conditions are not right for the grass. The soil may be compacted, waterlogged, hungry, or too acidic, or the site may be too shady. To control moss effectively, identify and eliminate the cause.

MORE MAGIC CARPETS

If you want to try something different, you could grow a wildflower meadow or a fragrant carpet of herbs. Low-growing chamomile and thyme lawns smell absolutely delicious but will not, however, withstand heavy use or football games. Unlike grass, they do not need mowing, but they do need careful hand-weeding, so maintenance is time-consuming.

Head
for the border

Trees, shrubs, and flowers of all kinds have a role to play in your organic garden. Not only do they provide a beautiful display to please the eye, they can also provide natural habitats for wildlife.

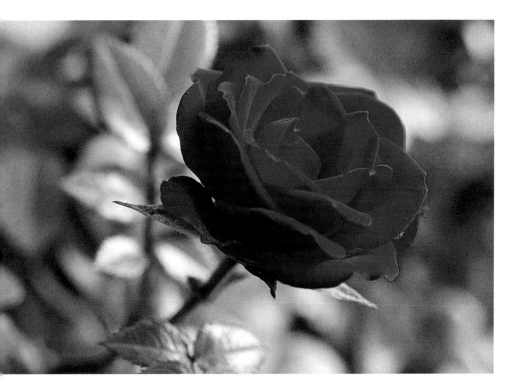

In addition to providing stunning visual appeal, the presence of a rich variety of plants in your garden can actually increase the overall diversity of the garden and provide an environment that is of benefit to birds, insects, and other types of wildlife, too.

You could try growing scented flowers, herbs, and foliage to add another sensory dimension to your garden. To enjoy the perfumes of these plants to the full, grow them in a place where you can brush against them to release their scent. There are many types of vegetable that can also add another level of interest, having aesthetic as well as edible appeal. You can grow them either interspersed among other plants in your borders or in a separate vegetable patch designed for beauty as well as function. Know your limitations – choose

Work with nature and nature will work

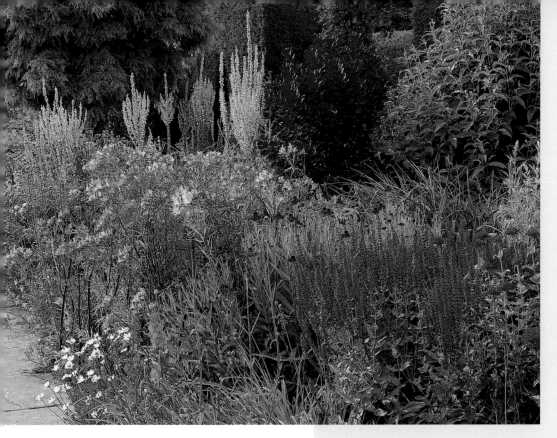

HEAD FOR THE BORDER

plants that suit your site and soil, and that fit the space available. The barriers and control methods that are suitable for preventing pests in a vegetable garden may not be visually appealing in an ornamental garden, so you may need to consider using some of the alternative methods suggested for promoting plant health and controlling pests and diseases.

All plants will benefit from careful soil preparation before planting. Weed the whole area thoroughly, paying particular attention to the removal of deep-rooted perennial weeds. Add some bulky organic material to improve the structure of your soil and to provide enough nutrients. Water thoroughly at planting, and remember to continue to water frequently until the plants are established.

with you.

DICK KITTO, *COMPOSTING*, 1984

TREES & SHRUBS

These add height to a garden and create a permanent framework as well as providing shade and a variety of habitats that attract birds and other wildlife.

Organic growing tips

❖ Use loose or fabric mulch to control weeds when the plants are young

❖ Remove dead, damaged, or diseased parts promptly

❖ Prune to encourage flowering, and to control size and shape where appropriate

HEDGES

A filter for wind and noise, hedges create shelter for tender plants and provide food and shelter for wildlife.

Organic growing tips

❖ Choose native species for maximum wildlife benefit

❖ Use loose or fabric mulch to control weeds when the plants are young

❖ Avoid disturbing nesting birds by not pruning in spring

❖ Allow leaves to gather at the bottom of the hedge to provide a wildlife habitat

HERBACEOUS PERENNIALS

Available to suit all soils and situations, they produce seeds for birds in autumn, provide hibernation sites for insects, and produce nectar and pollen that attract bees, butterflies, and beneficial insects.

Organic growing tips

❖ Lift and divide clumps every three to four years to avoid congestion

❖ Use loose mulches for weed control and water retention

❖ Leave stems and seed heads standing through the winter for wildlife benefit and to provide visual interest

ANNUALS

These come in a wide range to suit all soils and situations and flower for only one year, thus offering a quick way to provide changing color in the garden. They may self-seed in some cases, returning the following year without any need for resowing. The nectar and pollen that they produce attracts bees, butterflies, and beneficial insects.

Organic growing tips

❖ Weed thoroughly before sowing or planting

❖ Hand-weed or hoe during the early stages of growth

❖ Allow the seeds to form after flowering to encourage self-seeding

Good enough to eat

The taste of fresh organic vegetables, taken straight from the garden to the kitchen, has to be experienced to be fully appreciated. Growing your own produce is very satisfying, great fun, and definitely healthy.

When you grow your own vegetables, you have the peace of mind of knowing exactly how they have been produced, and can choose your favorite crops and varieties, including unusual ones not easily found in stores. Best of all, anyone can do it. You do not need to be an expert, nor have a huge garden to grow food. Many vegetables can be grown among your flowers and shrubs, appreciated for their appearance as well as their edible qualities. Even if you do not have a garden at all, window boxes, pots, or organic growing bags can produce herbs, salads, and some vegetables.

THE CHOICE IS YOURS
It is much better to start small and succeed than to get disheartened because you cannot manage to look after a huge plot. Be realistic about how much time and energy you can actually devote to growing vegetables. Decide what you and your family like to eat. There is no point in growing row after row of fantastic radishes, for instance, if no one is going to touch them.

Many gardening catalogues supply organically grown seeds, and sometimes plants too (*see page 238*). Others supply seeds that, while not organic, will at least not have been treated with pesticides after harvest. Organic gardening groups are a good source of information about the local availability of organic seeds and plants.

Most vegetables grow best in a sheltered, sunny position, but some, such as beets and spinach, do well in partial shade. If you do not have suitable conditions at home, or need more space, it may be worth thinking about renting an allotment.

Once you've bitten into your first home-grown, sun-ripened

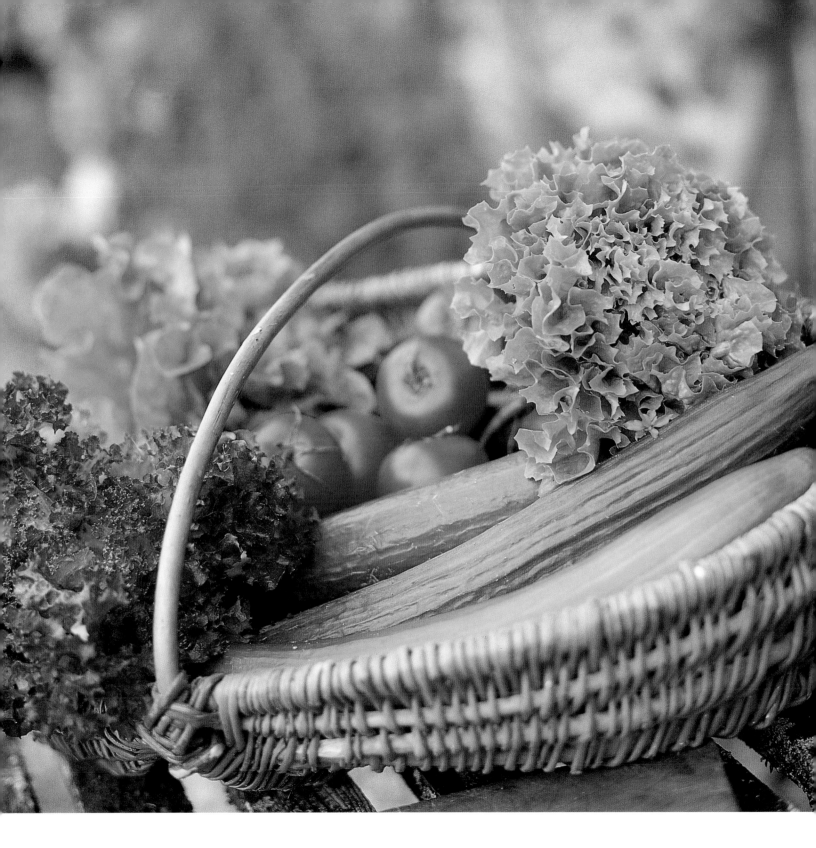

tomato, fresh from the vine, you'll be hooked.

PAULINE PEARS, HDRA – THE ORGANIC ORGANISATION

Good enough to eat

WINTER GREENS

✤ Land cress – similar to watercress, very hardy, strong flavor

✤ Winter purslane – mild flavor, succulent leaves, flowers also edible

✤ Mizuna – peppery flavor, deeply cut leaves

✤ Giant red mustard – hot flavor, moderately hardy

✤ Mache – mild flavor; leaves and flowers edible

SUMMER SALADS

✤ Arugula – strong, peppery flavor

✤ Bibb leaf lettuce – mild flavor, many different varieties

✤ Cress – strong, hot flavor, quick-growing

✤ Endive and chicory – slightly bitter flavor, many different varieties

✤ Leaf radish – special variety that produces leafy growth rather than roots, similar flavor to the usual radishes

GETTING A GOOD START

Root crops should be sown directly into their growing position. Most other hardy crops can either be sown direct or given a head start by sowing in pots or trays indoors. Tender crops, however, will need to be started off indoors. You can also buy young plants that are ready for transplanting. Some organically grown ones are now available (*see page 238*).

FROM THE GARDEN TO THE TABLE

Make sure you provide seedlings and transplants with enough water at the beginning. After that, if the soil has good structure, most crops should not need extra water in normal conditions. Keep your plants free from weeds by regular hand-weeding and hoeing, especially in the early stages. Most crops taste best when young and tender, so harvest just as they reach maturity and enjoy them as soon as possible.

EASY LEAVES ALL YEAR ROUND

Harvesting a regular supply of fresh, organic green leaves from your garden throughout the year is a simple matter of planning.

Summer leaves are so easy to grow and come in some delicious varieties (*see left*). Seeds should be sown from late spring to mid-summer, resowing every three to four weeks for a continuous supply of leaves. Sow thickly in shallow drills, up to 1¼ in (3 cm) deep and 4–6 in (10–15 cm) wide, and

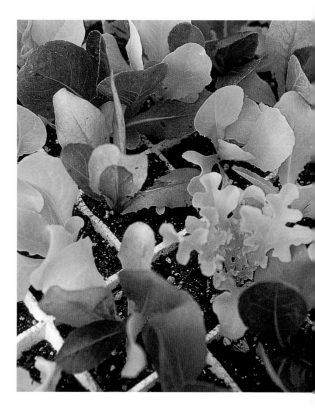

harvest when about 4 in (10 cm) high. The leaves can be harvested with scissors or a sharp knife, then left to grow back two to three times. You can also grow some delicious salad herbs (*see far right*).

Fresh greens are particularly welcome in winter. Many (*see above left*) are good in salads, stir-fries, or soups. Sow them directly into the soil in late summer, then thin the seedlings to the required spacing specified on the packet. These plants will survive until late autumn and some will last right through to spring in a mild winter. It is best to provide protective covers in bad weather.

FIRST–TIME VEGETABLES

Here we suggest a selection of vegetables for the novice vegetable gardener. They will usually produce good results in most soils, do not need any special techniques or equipment, and can all be sown or planted directly into your garden.

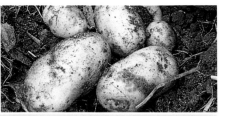

VEGETABLE	PLANT/SOW	HARVEST	COMMENTS
Beets	spring – early summer	summer – autumn	harvest early crops when still small; later varieties store well; red, yellow, and even striped varieties available
Lima beans	spring or autumn	summer	may need support when fully grown; harvest young for the best flavor; good for freezing; some varieties are suitable for sowing in autumn
Chard or leaf beet	spring – summer	all year round	hardy enough to survive most winters from a late sowing; spinachlike flavor; available in a range of stem colors
Zucchini	early summer	late summer – early autumn	cover the seeds with a plastic bottle or cloche to speed their germination; harvest regularly when the fruits form; plants die with the first frost; green, yellow, round, and long varieties available
Garlic	autumn or spring	late summer	plant individual cloves; harvest when the leaves start to turn yellow; stores well when dry
Leeks	spring	late summer – early spring	sow close together, transplanting when pencil-thick; some varieties are very hardy; attractive varieties with blue-tinged leaves available
Lettuce	early spring – summer	early summer – autumn	sow a small amount every two to three weeks for a continuous supply of lettuce throughout the summer; a wide range of types, flavors and colors available
Onions or shallots from sets	early spring or autumn	early summer – late summer	plant with the tips just below the surface of the soil and watch out for birds tweaking them out; harvest when the leaves have fallen over; red, white, and yellow varieties available
Potatoes	spring	summer – early autumn	early, maincrop and salad varieties are all available; protect the young leaves from frost; harvest when the leaves die back; maincrop varieties store well in cool, dark conditions
Radishes	spring – late summer	early summer – early autumn	sow a few every two to three weeks for a continuous supply throughout the summer, harvest young for the best flavor; need moist soil to do well

SUMMER SALAD HERBS FOR CONTAINERS

❧ Chervil – delicate, ferny leaf, mild anise flavor

❧ Cilantro – harvest young to prevent seeds forming

❧ Nasturtium – peppery flavor, flowers and leaves edible, tumbling habit good for baskets

❧ Dill – feathery gray-green leaves, traditionally used with fish

❧ Basil – comes in a range of sizes, colors, and flavors, a "must" for tomato salads and pesto

❧ Summer savory – leaves and flowers edible, good with fresh or dried beans

Grow these even if you try nothing else. All can be used raw in salads, or added to soups and sauces where they enhance summer cooking with fresh, distinctive flavors. Sow from late spring to mid-summer or buy young plants. Use a general-purpose organic potting compost and make sure that your container has good drainage. Provide adequate water to prevent them setting seed prematurely.

Fruits of success

Growing organic fruit brings great satisfaction and is a luxury we can all afford. Your efforts will be rewarded with crops of delicious fruit.

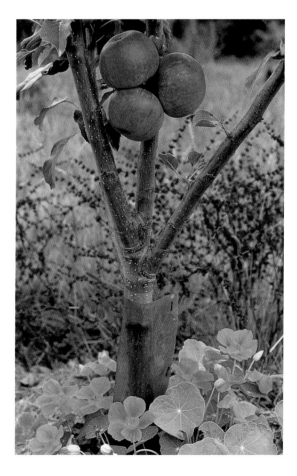

It takes a little bit of time to grow fruit but, within a couple of years of planting, you will be able to harvest sweet, succulent organic fruit for eating fresh and for turning into mouth-watering pies, tarts, and other desserts. Some fruits can be carefully stored for winter, while others can be frozen to provide fruit out of season, or made into delicious jams and chutneys.

FAVORABLE CONDITIONS

Fruit trees and bushes are going to be in the ground for a long time, so they need a fertile soil that will retain moisture but not get waterlogged. If your soil is less than perfect, you can improve it by adding bulky organic material not just to the planting hole, but to the whole surrounding area. Remove all perennial weeds and mulch after planting to prevent weeds returning and to help retain moisture. Water your plants well when they are first planted and continue to water them in dry periods for the first couple of years.

The best site will be as sunny as possible. Although some fruit can tolerate shady sites, most grow best in full sun. Shelter is also important. Strong winds can cause damage, and discourage pollinating insects at flowering time. Hedges make excellent windbreaks, but you may need to put up temporary barriers while they become established.

YOUR NATURAL ALLIES

Beneficial creatures are welcome in the organic fruit garden to help with pest control. Attract them by growing a range of flowering plants in among the tree and bushes (*see page 160*).

SPACE – THE NONEXISTENT FRONTIER

You do not need a huge garden to grow fruit. Modern varieties of fruit are quite compact, which makes it possible to include tree and bush fruit in even the smallest of gardens. Fruit trees and bushes can also be grown against walls and fences as cordons and espaliers, making attractive screens to divide a garden in addition to providing delicious fruit. Dwarf varieties and unusual containers further broaden the range of possibilities (*see page 174*).

Nothing beats the joy of growing your own organic fruit.

JACKIE GEAR, EXECUTIVE DIRECTOR, HDRA – THE ORGANIC ORGANISATION

Fruits of success

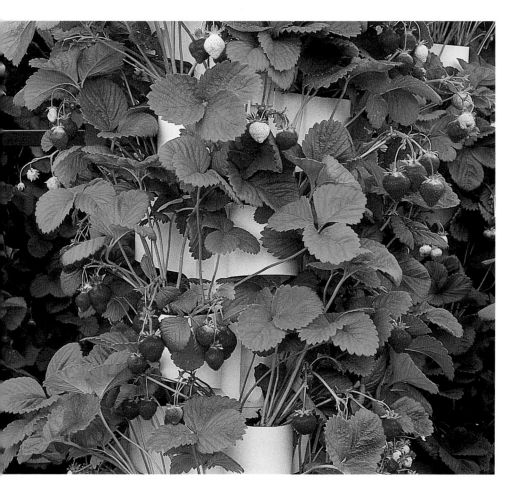

5–6½ ft (1.5–2 m), and produce up to a dozen fruits each year. Little pruning is required, but you must be careful to water your trees regularly to ensure the fruits do not split while they are growing. Plant your peach tree in a general-purpose organic potting mix. Provide good drainage at the bottom of the pot, and change the potting mix each year in autumn. Leave your tree outdoors until autumn, bringing it under cover soon after leaf drop until late winter or early spring where temperatures drop well below freezing.

A TOWER OF STRAWBERRIES

Who would say no to a steady stream of delicious organic strawberries from their garden – even if they do not actually have a garden? This space-saving method makes it possible. Strawberries grow well in half an old barrel or in a specially designed "tower", where the fruit dangle enticingly over the edge. This method keeps the strawberries out of the way of slugs, and makes them easy to protect from birds. Plant them in organic potting mix in the summer, leaving them outside through winter since they need cold temperatures to develop properly. When spring comes, place the strawberries in a sunny position and water regularly. If using a tower, make sure the plants at the bottom get plenty of water, too. To prevent disease buildup, start with new plants every year.

PEACHES IN A POT

What could be nicer than an elegant little potful of blossoms in spring followed by a mini-harvest of succulent home-grown peaches? Varieties of naturally dwarf peaches are perfect for growing in pots and will look good in a garden, in a sunny little courtyard, or even on a city roof terrace. When fully grown they will reach about

EASY-TO-GROW FRUITS

Here are some suggestions for fruits you can grow yourself. They are quite easy to produce, although do follow the tips (*see right*). Potential growing forms are also given, such as cordons (in which the plant is trained as a single main stem against wires or a fence) and espaliers (where the plant is trained flat against wires or a fence on a main stem with branches on either side).

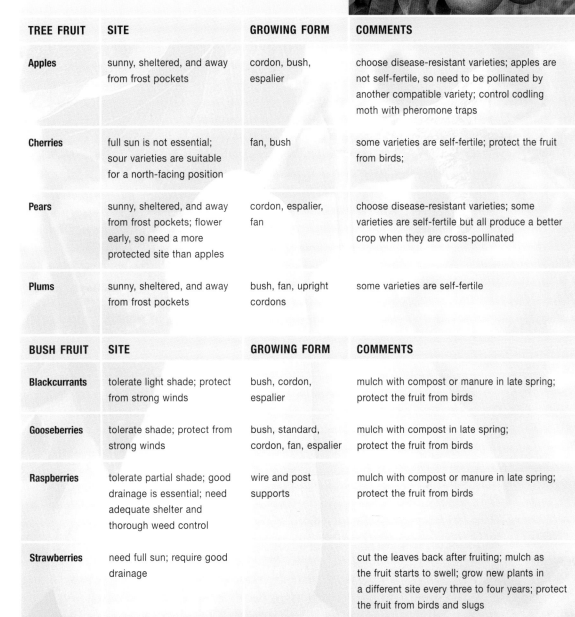

TREE FRUIT	SITE	GROWING FORM	COMMENTS
Apples	sunny, sheltered, and away from frost pockets	cordon, bush, espalier	choose disease-resistant varieties; apples are not self-fertile, so need to be pollinated by another compatible variety; control codling moth with pheromone traps
Cherries	full sun is not essential; sour varieties are suitable for a north-facing position	fan, bush	some varieties are self-fertile; protect the fruit from birds;
Pears	sunny, sheltered, and away from frost pockets; flower early, so need a more protected site than apples	cordon, espalier, fan	choose disease-resistant varieties; some varieties are self-fertile but all produce a better crop when they are cross-pollinated
Plums	sunny, sheltered, and away from frost pockets	bush, fan, upright cordons	some varieties are self-fertile

BUSH FRUIT	SITE	GROWING FORM	COMMENTS
Blackcurrants	tolerate light shade; protect from strong winds	bush, cordon, espalier	mulch with compost or manure in late spring; protect the fruit from birds
Gooseberries	tolerate shade; protect from strong winds	bush, standard, cordon, fan, espalier	mulch with compost in late spring; protect the fruit from birds
Raspberries	tolerate partial shade; good drainage is essential; need adequate shelter and thorough weed control	wire and post supports	mulch with compost or manure in late spring; protect the fruit from birds
Strawberries	need full sun; require good drainage		cut the leaves back after fruiting; mulch as the fruit starts to swell; grow new plants in a different site every three to four years; protect the fruit from birds and slugs

TIPS ON FRUIT-GROWING

❖ Tree fruits that grow well outside include apples, pears, plums, and cherries

❖ Less-hardy fruits such as peaches, apricots, grapes, and figs may need some protection

❖ Currants and berries produce plentiful harvests for many years; many are tolerant of harsher conditions than tree fruit and are quicker to start producing crops

❖ Both tree and bush fruit can be trained in attractive ways, providing visual as well as edible appeal

❖ Choose varieties that are less susceptible to diseases and pests where possible

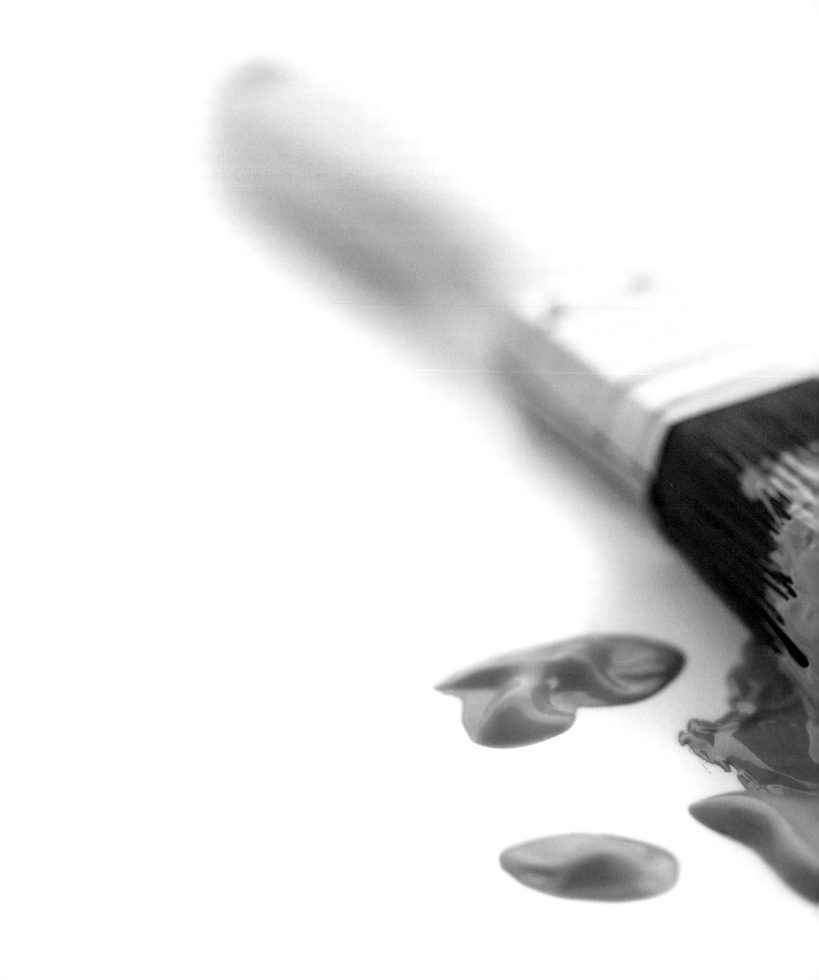

organic
HOME & OFFICE

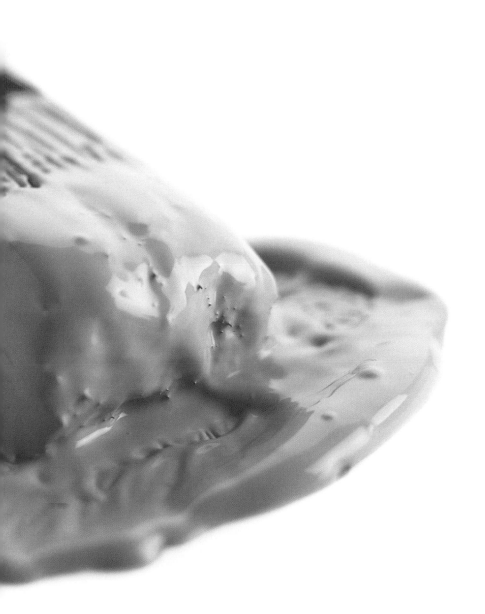

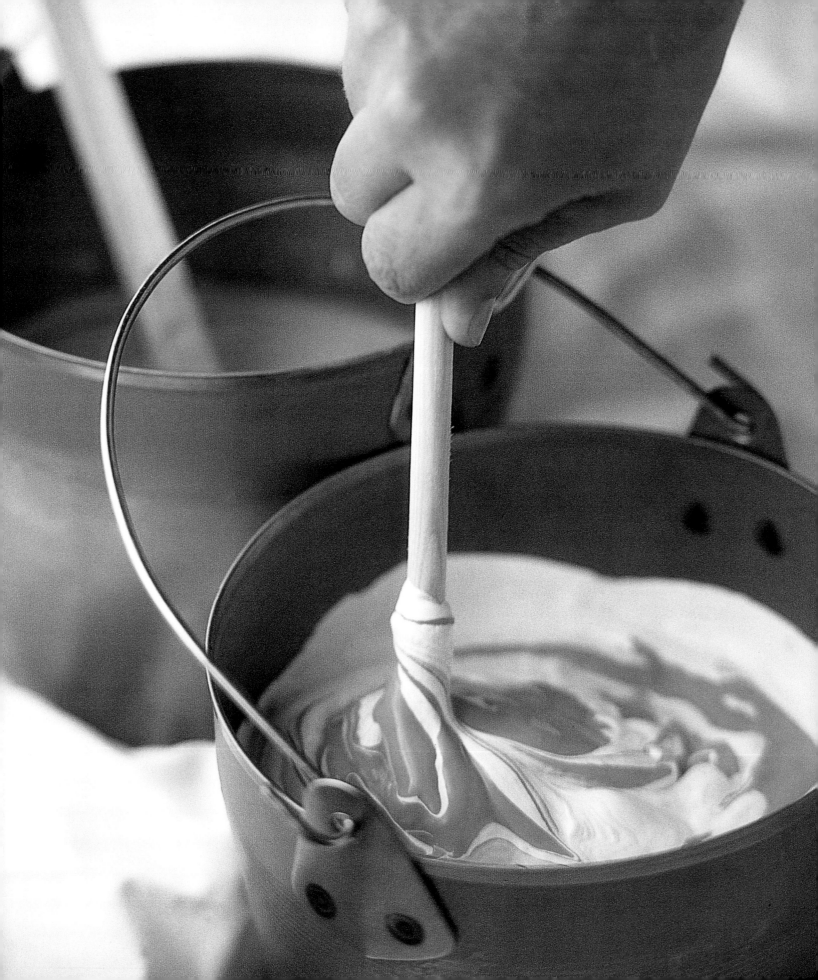

WHY GO organic

The route to global survival, through equity and sustainability, is marked by lifestyle changes, small and large, dramatic and subtle, and by technical fixes, radical solutions, and practical compromises at home and at work.

Since the Industrial Revolution, Western consumer society has progressed along an unsustainable path that everyone else in the world seems drawn to follow. There are a number of ways, however, in which each of us can contribute to reducing the environmental impact of our homes and lifestyles by making considered consumer choices and by choosing sustainable, eco-friendly options.

GLOBAL SOLUTIONS

We have all witnessed the darker consequences of the modern consumer society: the contamination of the air, earth, and water, the poisoning of our own bodies by barely restrained pollution and the plunder of not just our own environment, but that of the rest of the world. The environmental answer to these problems can be summed up in two words: equity – the fair distribution of the earth's resources among its peoples – and sustainability – the use and replenishment of resources at a rate that does not deplete natural

supplies. If we can consume less and we can use sustainable alternatives, these aims can be achieved. In the home and office this means maximum energy conservation and efficiency – using insulation and efficient boilers, for example, and replacing fossil fuels with renewable energy sources such as solar power.

GOING ORGANIC IN THE HOME & OFFICE

There are many simple things that all of us can do to make a start on the road to sustainability, based on our day-to-day behavior and our choices as consumers. For example, rather than buying all your food and household goods from the supermarket, why not explore local, sustainable options? When making purchases of all kinds, make informed choices and look for eco-friendly alternatives. And at the end of a product's life, seek methods of recycling. These ideas, as well as those for using energy and resources more responsibly, can also be applied to our working environments.

Choose eco-friendly or recyclable alternatives such as long-life light bulbs

Make sure that electrical equipment is turned off when not in use

Try to recycle whenever you can

Use sustainable materials and renewable energy sources at home

Recycle your office's waste paper and photocopier cartridges

Your questions answered

You want to live in an eco-friendly home – where do you start? Each time you buy a product for your home or office ask yourself these questions: What is it made of? Where does it come from? How does it work?

How do I know whether something is organic?

Look at the labels (*see page 246*). When buying timber look for the Forest Stewardship Council (FSC) logo or other certification. On other goods, a fair trade logo may mean they are environmentally friendly, but does not guarantee organic production (*see page 220*). Look for labels of organic certification bodies and efficiency rating on electrical goods.

How do I make a "green" home?

This is much easier than you might think. Every time something in your house needs replacing or improving, there will be an eco-friendly alternative for you to choose to gradually make your house a bit "greener". From insulation to draft-proofing, flooring to paint, there are organic products or methods of recycling that can help.

How do I run a "green" office or business?

The benefits of an energy-efficient workplace can also contribute to the profitability of a business. Obey the general rule: reduce, reuse, recycle (*see page 182*). Switch off electrical equipment rather than leaving it on standby. And if you are looking to improve the environmental performance of your business, get advice from a local energy advice organization.

Do eco-friendly products cost more?

Sometimes, but not if you consider the cost to the environment. Small eco-friendly producers are often unable to match the economies of scale of larger companies, so their products are not as cheap. The more we buy eco-friendly products, however, the bigger the demand will be and the cheaper products will become. Paying out more initially can save you money over time, too – with solar panels for water heating, for example.

Can I buy renewable energy?

Yes. This is getting easier than it used to be. Some local electricity suppliers now operate "green" tariffs under which you can pay a small premium to ensure your electricity comes from a renewable source or supports the development of renewables (*see page 197*). In some countries you can buy your electricity from a company which specializes in electricity from renewable sources.

What does sustainable mean?

Sustainability is the practice of methods of living and working which do not deplete the planet's resources – whether those resources are minerals, fossil fuels, plant and animal species, or the air we breathe and the water that ensures the continuance of life. In essence, being sustainable means taking out only what we can put back in.

What is sustainable forestry?

Sustainable forestry is a system ensuring well-managed forests that conform to environmental criteria including the protection of biodiversity, water resources, and soil structure (*see page 190*). As well as social considerations, sustainable forestry also recognizes the land rights of indigenous peoples.

Where can I learn about eco-friendly building?

One source of information is the US Green Building Council. The USGBC is a nonprofit consensus coaltion of the building industry that promotes eco-friendly policies. Similar associations are listed internationally on the internet – try searching under "environmental" or "alternative building".

Where can I go if I want to ask more questions?

Look in the directory at the back of this book (*see page 222*) to find lots of contacts who can help you to live and work organically. If you have a general question about where to go next, try one of the nonprofit organizations in this book's directory. Many have a comprehensive directory of environmental organizations, consultants, companies, and visitor centers, as well as details of books and courses.

Where can I buy recycled products?

You can find recycled products in your local resale shops (Salvation Army stores, for instance), and health food stores. Look out for eco-friendly catalogues and other mail order or online specialist environmental group catalogues (*see page 223*), many of which are available on the internet.

Reduce and recycle

Many of the earth's resources are finite, and these are disappearing at an alarming rate. To create a sustainable planet we need to reduce the pollution we create and stop squandering the earth's natural reserves.

We are using irreplaceable fossil fuels and precious nonrenewable materials to manufacture endless products and materials. The burning of fossil fuels, and use of chemicals, and other toxic materials in manufacturing processes, is also causing huge pollution problems.

As well as the obvious problems in manufacturing and transporting goods, we are also creating huge waste problems

The golden rules of reducing waste are the three R's: Reduce, Reuse, and Recycle.

when we throw them away. Most trash that is not reused or recycled goes to landfill sites. These are unsightly, smelly, environmentally damaging places, and are rapidly becoming full. We need to reduce the volume of trash we send to landfill sites. Fortunately, this is possible, and it is perfectly feasible to reduce domestic trash by 90 percent.

less trash

The first step is to try to reduce the amount of waste you create in the first place. This can range from lifestyle choices such as resisting the temptation to buy things you do not need, to practical steps such as choosing products with less packaging, carrying your own reusable shopping bag, and buying in bulk. Reuse things or repair them where

possible. With a bit of imagination things can often be reused as something else rather than being thrown away. Recycle everything you cannot reuse: cans, glass, paper, fabrics, and some plastics.

We can also recycle organic waste. Organic waste is a problem in landfill sites as it cannot break down properly. Composting it returns the vital nutrients to the soil, turning a waste problem into a practical environmental solution (*see page 152*).

We all happily take our bottles, cans, and newspapers to be recycled, but seem to be less confident about recycling plastics – probably because recycling facilities for plastics have not been widely available, and possibly because there are so many different types of plastic in use. Most plastic materials are now number coded to make recycling easier.

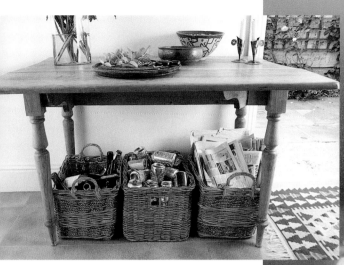

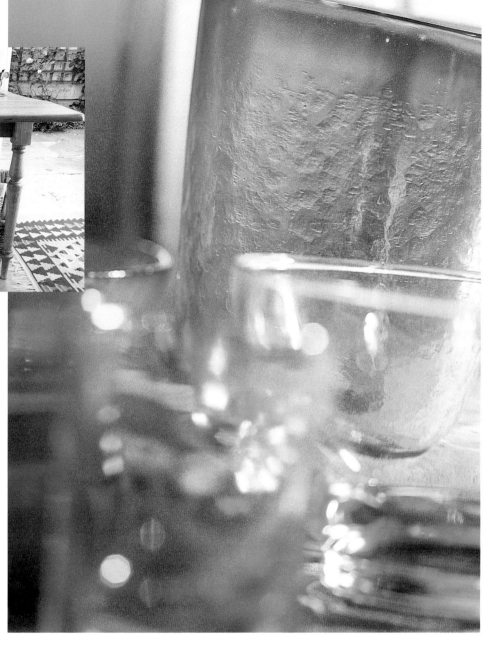

The type of plastic recycling facilities offered by local authorities varies. Some have plastic "banks" that will take any type of plastic. Other banks will only accept polyethylene terephthalate (PET) bottles, which can be recycled indefinitely, while others collect all the different types separately.

use recycled

Of course, for recycling to work there has to be a market for products made from recycled materials, so try to actively choose to buy them too. This not only supports the economics of recycling but also reduces our use of raw materials and the amount of pollution created.

Happily, there is a huge range of recycled products available, from electrical equipment to toilet paper. All paper products, both for the home and the office, are now widely available in recycled versions. There are also increasing numbers of recycled glass

and plastic products available. Plastic is even made into fleece clothing by the Patagonia clothing company (*see page 203*).

In the office all the general recycling rules apply, but there are some specific challenges. Help people in the office to separate out their trash by having clearly marked and easily used containers for

the different types of trash. Electronic equipment can usually be recycled, and ink cartridges can often be returned to the manufacturer for refilling. Paper is usually the biggest waste stream and incoming resource to offices. By using both sides – recycling it *and* buying recycled paper, you can help close the loop.

A clean sweep

Thanks to increasing public awareness of environmental issues, just about any chemical cleaning product will now have an "eco" alternative, from laundry detergents to dishwashing liquids, and bathroom cleaners.

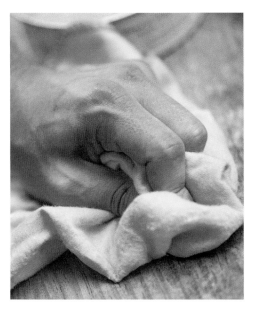

A look in most households' kitchen cupboards will reveal a range of different cleaning, washing, and pest-control products, often made up of unfamiliar chemicals. Where our predecessors would have used vinegar, beeswax, or plant-based soaps, we now have "modern" chemical cleaning products, many of which are petroleum-based and contain phosphates, organochlorines, and synthetic perfumes and colorings. With this cocktail of chemicals being flushed down our drains, plants, wildlife, and the human population suffer the effects. However, as public awareness of environmental issues has grown, demand has increased for a range of eco-friendly cleaning and washing products. Initially only found in health and healthfood stores, many of these products have now made their way onto the supermarket shelves.

alternatives

Choosing these products is a good place to start. There are many "natural" alternatives which predate commercial products, such as vinegar and water to clean windows or remove lime scale, and lemon juice to polish brass and silver. A general cream cleaner may do for both the kitchen and the bathroom. Where you do need to use detergents, use them in moderation.

Reducing your use of chemical products will make your house a safer place and benefit the wider environment.

Many eco-friendly cleaning products work just as well as their conventional alternatives. One of the most popular ranges is produced by Ecover, a Belgian company. Some shops buy products in bulk and will then decant products into the container you return to them, meaning less packaging and less waste.

labeling

As companies become aware that labeling their products as biodegradable or environmentally friendly could be a favorable selling point, it becomes more difficult for the consumer to establish which products are truly "green". The European Union (EU) Ecolabeling program is taking a step towards solving this problem. The program reduces the confusion by using Life Cycle Analysis. This looks at every stage in the manufacture, use, and disposal of a product, to identify those which do less damage to the environment. Currently, the only household cleaning products for which EU Ecolabel criteria have been developed are laundry detergents and dishwasher detergents, but criteria for floor cleaners and other cleaning products are under development.

pest control

Cleaning products are not the only chemicals in use around the house – we also use fly sprays, mouse poisons, head lice controls, and flea powders. While effective at killing the pests, they are likely to be hazardous to human health too. Where nonchemical alternatives can be used instead, they should be. Conventional mouse traps or ones that catch the mice live are just as effective as poisons and will not pass poisons on up the food chain. Conditioner and a comb for head lice are just as effective as chemical lice shampoos.

THE DIFFERENCES THAT COUNT

❖ Eco-friendly cleaning products use natural, vegetable-based cleaners that break down more quickly and more completely than petroleum-based detergents

❖ Alternative, eco-friendly products will not have been tested on animals

❖ Eco-friendly alternatives do not contain phosphates, which affect the nutrient balance of water life

❖ Enzymes (which can be irritants and cause asthmatic reactions) are not used in eco-friendly cleaning products

❖ Cleaning products that are eco-friendly do not contain optical bleaches (which can cause mutations in micro-organisms) or organochlorines (which can be toxic and carcinogenic)

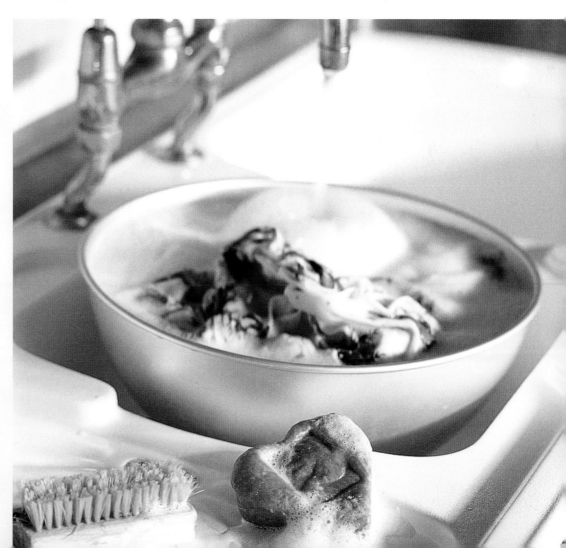

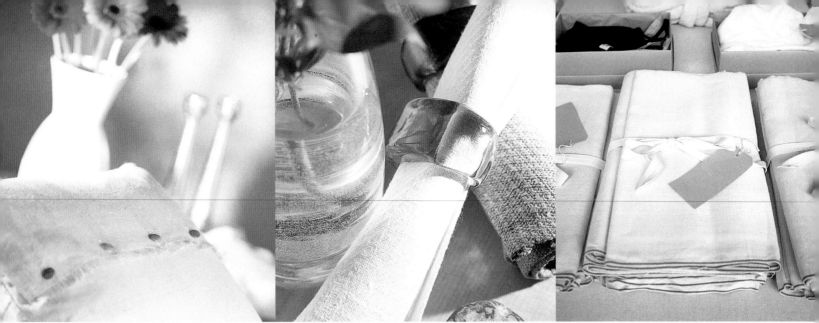

Into.
the interior

There are a number of golden rules you should follow to help you make environmentally friendly choices – whatever the product. Some of these are technical fixes, some are lifestyle choices.

The impact on the environment of our homes and offices is significant. Often we think of environmental damage as being done by industry. But among those industries are the domestic building and household product sectors in which we, as consumers, play a huge part. The more we try to make some lifestyle changes, the more we will reduce our impact on the planet.

We can work towards using less of the world's resources by cutting down on the amount we buy and use, and by choosing products and materials that are environmentally friendly. This includes looking at the raw materials used, the energy involved in manufacture, transportation and use, and what will happen to the products when their useful life is over.

One method of assessing this environmental impact is Life Cycle Analysis (LCA), which takes a "cradle-to-grave" approach. At the moment the tools for measuring LCAs are crude and full analyses have not been carried out for every product, nor is there full agreement on methodology for doing LCAs. However, it is worth bearing in mind as a general concept. More

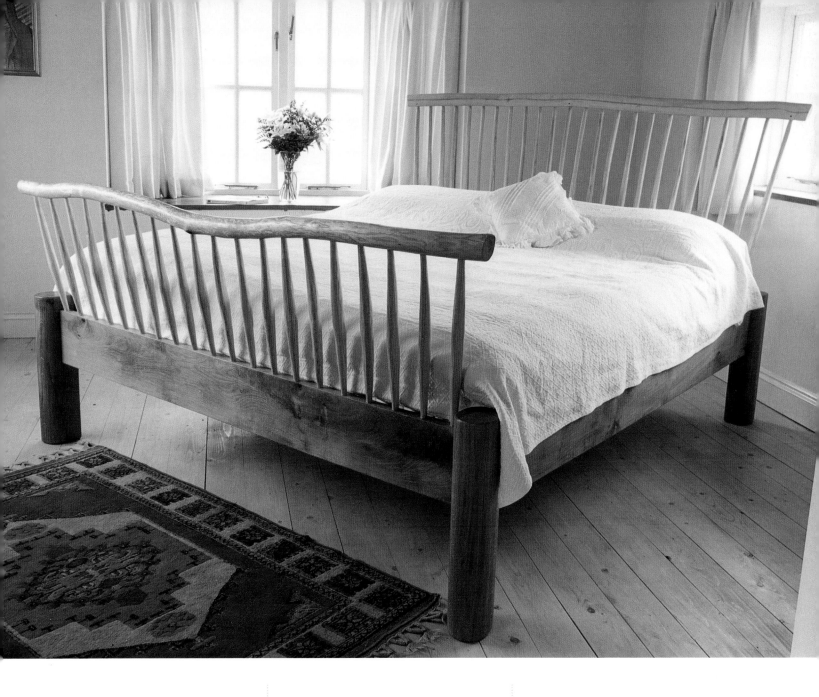

information is needed to make a reasoned judgement, and a number of certification programs can help this.

furniture

There is a wide range of furniture made with the least environmental impact possible: from hand-crafted pieces made from reclaimed or sustainably grown timbers such as teak, sycamore, and cherry to upholstered furniture using 100 percent organic fibers. A certification mark on wooden furniture and household products will ensure that the wood comes from managed woodlands rather than from endangered forests (*see page 190*).

Into. the interior

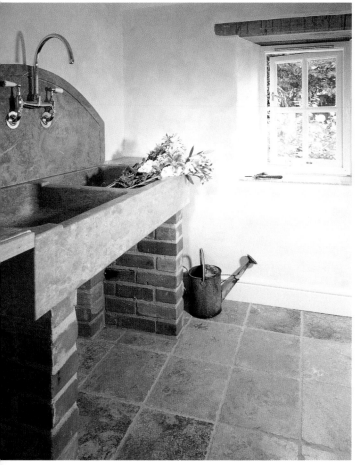

flooring

Most environmentally friendly products used for flooring are also aesthetically pleasing – terracotta tiles, coir matting, cork floors, and even linoleum, which is made of totally natural materials. Companies such as Crucial Trading and Fired Earth stock a wide range of natural floorings. As a bonus, with any of the above you will lessen any allergy problems caused by dust mites. But if you really cannot live without carpet, the best options are wool and natural mixes that are unbleached and colored with natural dyes and have jute or burlap backing in place of foam.

fabric

You can deck every room of your house with eco-friendly fabrics , from the towels in your bathroom to the sheets on your bed, and from the napkins on the table to the cushions on your sofa. Though essentially a "natural" material, conventionally grown cotton is usually treated with vast amounts of artificial pesticides and herbicides (*see page 204*). The alternative is organically grown, unbleached cotton or other materials such as hemp or wool. Items labeled "easy care" or "noniron" may have had their fibers treated with formaldehyde, so avoid these when you can. Choose undyed, unbleached products and, if you cannot find unbleached, look for those bleached with hydrogen peroxide rather than chlorine bleaches. For comforters and pillows, buy natural down or feather rather than polyester-filled.

health

Recent years have seen a huge growth of interest in the relationship between health and buildings. Sick Building Syndrome and the increase in allergies, medical hypersensitivity, and asthma – notably in children – have spurred this on. We are all too often subjected to an unhealthy environment, living in houses that contain hundreds of different chemicals in everything from the insulation in the roof to the food we eat; we are exposed to external air and water pollutants; we make and are subjected to incessant noise – all of which may lead to health problems.

power

As the number of electrical appliances in the average household increases, so does the amount of power that we use – usually from fossil-fuel power stations that contribute to global warming. A few

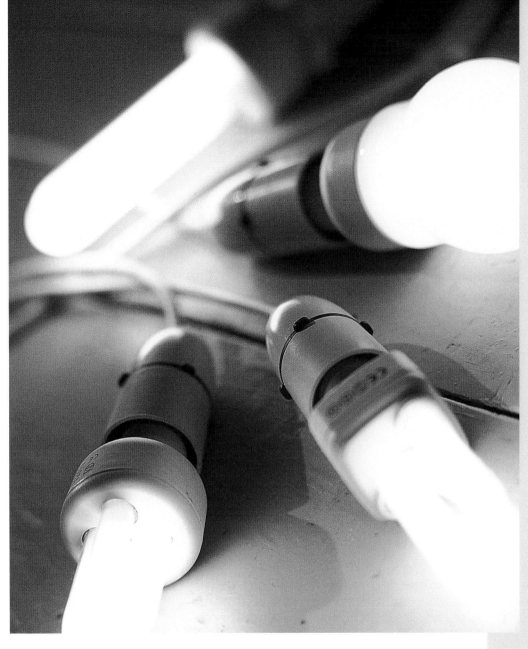

ENERGY-SAVING IDEAS

❖ **Avoid** putting more water in the pot than you need.

❖ **Use a clothes line** where possible, rather than a tumble drier.

❖ **Boil water** for cooking in a tea kettle first, since it is more efficient than the stove-top and saves energy.

❖ **Use a toaster** – it is more efficient than your grill and does not waste heat.

❖ **Avoid** using battery-powered appliances. A wind-up radio gives you half an hour of power for only 25 seconds of winding. Buy a wind-up watch instead of a battery-powered watch.

❖ **Use** a dynamo-powered light when out on your bike at night, or flashing light-emitting diode (LED) lights, which are the most efficient and use the smallest batteries.

❖ **Opt** for rechargeable batteries if you cannot avoid batteries altogether. But do not use them in smoke alarms as they run down suddenly. Be careful when disposing of batteries – ask your local authority if they have a collection point.

❖ **Save water** by making sure that you do not leave taps running, and take showers rather than baths. Install a low-flush toilet (which can save up to 90 per-cent of your flushing water) or divert rainwater for toilet flushing.

simple steps can reduce your power consumption. Energy-efficient (compact fluorescent) light bulbs, though more expensive initially than conventional light bulbs, will last longer and save money on your electricity bills. Buy energy-efficient appliances and always look for efficiency ratings on household appliances like dishwashers, washing machines, and ranges to find the most efficient. However, while a double-door refrigerator may be efficient for its size it will use far more energy than a smaller one at a lower rating.

In the office, look closely at equipment you buy. The new liquid crystal display (LCD) monitors are compatible with all standard personal computers and a 15 in (38 cm) LCD screen uses much less energy than a standard cathode ray tube – typically 18 watts as opposed to approximately 200 watts.

Focus on wood

Although the depletion of our natural forests represents an ongoing environmental tragedy, there is a lot you can do to make sure that the wood you use in your home comes from sustainably managed forests.

Wood is infinitely flexible and adaptable. No other material can meet the requirements of so many different building elements, from structural support, flooring, doors, and windows, to decorative finishes and furniture. It is easily accessible to DIY enthusiasts and professional builders alike. And there are also environmental advantages to using timber, the most important being that it is a renewable resource. The value of our forests is incalculable. As climate change becomes established, what is left of the world's forests can be seen as an increasingly important reservoir of carbon dioxide, which would otherwise be released into the atmosphere. As well as effectively storing carbon dioxide, forests trap air pollution, prevent soil erosion, store and filter surface water, and support a multitude of plant and animal species.

Nonsustainable forestry worldwide is responsible for loss of biodiversity, clear-felling, monoculture, and damage to soil structure, not to mention the loss of local people's land rights. We are all familiar with the loss of tropical rainforests – currently being cleared at the rate of 142 million acres every year – but the felling of old-growth forests in northern hemisphere territories such as Canada, Scandinavia, and Russia is causing many of the same problems in their local environments.

forest futures

To counter these problems a genuinely independent certification system guaranteeing ecological sensitivity and sustainability was established in 1993. The Forest Stewardship Council (FSC) is a nonprofit organization whose membership comprises environmentalists, timber traders, indigenous peoples' organizations, community forestry groups, forest workers' unions, forestry professionals, and retail companies. The FSC is the only worldwide organization offering a credible timber certification scheme for all types of forest, and receives support from Friends of the Earth, the World Wide Fund for Nature (WWF), and Greenpeace among others. Certification is carried out by independent organizations that are accredited,

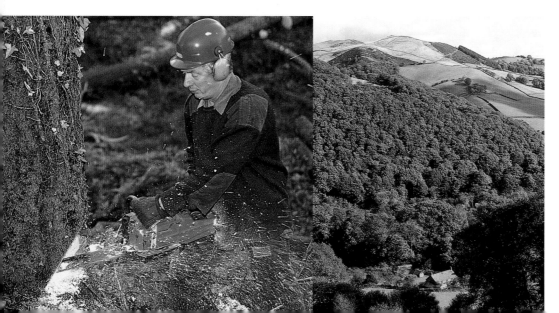

STAMP OF APPROVAL

The FSC publishes a set of criteria by which it judges certification, including environmental considerations such as the protection of biodiversity, water resources, and soil structure, and social considerations such as the rights of indigenous peoples and forestry workers. Regular inspections of forests and processing plants are carried out to maintain standards. There are currently nine certified forests in the UK, covering nearly 15,000 acres (6,000 hectares).

SUPPLIERS

A group of companies known as the 95+ Group and coordinated by the WWF, has pledged to meet certain targets on sourcing sustainably produced timber. Of the popular high-street names, Great Mills aim to stock *only* certified products by the end of 2000, Do It All plan to do the same by 2005, and B&Q reached 99.1 percent of its target of a 100 percent certified range of stock by early 2000.

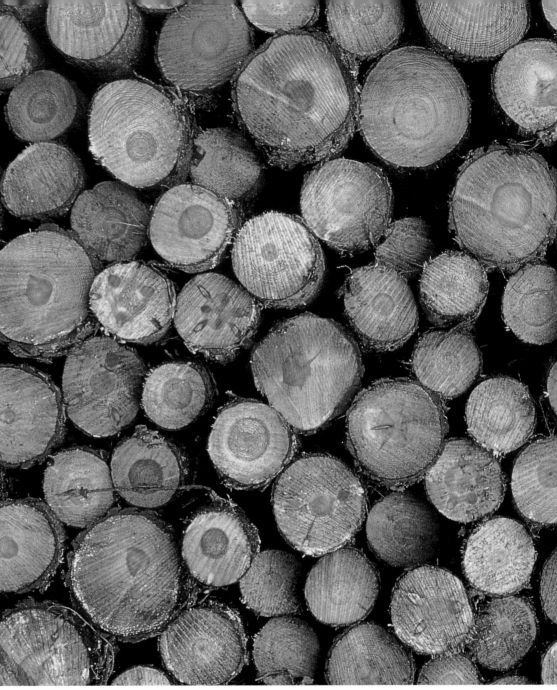

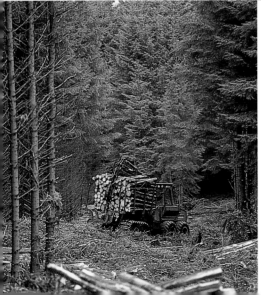

evaluated, and monitored by the FSC. Two certifiers have been accredited in the UK: the Société Générale de Surveillance (SGS) Forestry under its "Qualifor" program, and the Soil Association with its "Woodmark" program. The credibility of this program is enhanced by the Soil Association's experience of certifying organic farming and food. A wide range of forests has been certified to FSC standards, and many wood-based products from these, including paper, furniture, wallpaper, and various DIY materials are now available (*see above left*). Just shop wisely and look for accreditation symbols from certifiers on any timber and wood or paper products you buy.

Structurally
sound

So, if you have just bought or built your new house, and would like to make sure that it is a healthy environment to live and work in, how do you go about decorating an organic, eco-friendly environment?

There are as many choices of decorative finish in an eco-friendly building as there are conventional alternatives.

paints

Let's start with the walls. Normal practice is to use vinyl emulsion on walls and ceilings, and oil-based gloss on internal and external woodwork. But concerns about the effects on human health of exposure to volatile compounds (now labeled on paint cans as VOC content or rating) in such paints have led to them gradually being replaced by water-based vinyls. However, these may be more damaging to the environment in their production.

All paints and stains are either water- or solvent-based. Natural or organic paints and stains use plant-based dyes,

solvents, and fillers – renewable resources that will biodegrade. All solvents are designed to evaporate – this is how paint dries. Although some people do have an allergic response to the solvents in natural paints, this is far less common and serious than for petrochemical solvents. Another bonus with plant-based solvents is that they react with the natural oils and resins in untreated wood, creating a chemical bond and a breathable finish, rather than an impervious coating that is can crack and flake.

In an organic living space you have several options. Use unpainted finishes where possible, and instead of vinyls use limewash or mineral- or plant-based paints for walls and ceilings, and mineral masonry paint for outside. There are a variety of organic paints and stains,

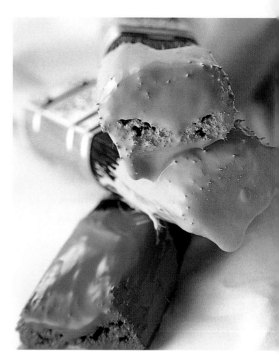

wood waxes, and linseed oils for use on internal and external woodwork. Paints produced by some companies, for example, are not solvent-based, have no

DIY

The same cautionary principles apply when buying other DIY products such as glues, adhesives, and building materials. Composite boards, such as medium-density fiberboard (MDF), may seem to save trees, but are a less human-friendly option. The majority of MDFs consist of very small pieces of wood glued together, and it is the glue that is usually the problem environmentally. Plywood is glued together using formaldehyde (a known animal and probable human carcinogen), and chipboard is glued together with urea-formaldehyde (which can cause skin irritation and breathing difficulties).

Look for the alternatives: softboard, mediumboard, and hardboard are all made by felting wood fibers and bonding them using heat and pressure. No synthetic glues are used.

insulation

If you are looking to insulate your attic or walls, there are a number of natural alternatives coming onto the market. Some alternatives are is made from surplus books, newspapers, and telephone directories. Sheep's wool is another possibility, and it is hoped that a wool insulation product will soon be available. Its insulation value is similar to that of mineral fibers. Also, it is slow to ignite and tends to melt away from any fire source and self-extinguish.

added lead, and are virtually odorless – and the cans are recyclable and reusable. Other companies make organic paints and varnishes using natural plant oils and waxes, plant-based solvents and earth and mineral pigments. Make sure to look, and ask for, eco-friendly paint and varnish brands.

Design for life

Whether you are designing a new house or office from scratch, adapting an existing property, or modernizing a listed building, eco-friendly options can open new doors and vistas.

When building your own house with organic living in mind, the most important decision is to choose a site that lends itself to sustainability. Once a house is built it can be remodeled, but you are stuck with your site. There are a number of features you should be looking for (many of which will apply when buying an existing property too).

Houses and offices should be designed with their end-users in mind – imagine a company of lawyers, dealing with confidential matters, finding themselves in an open plan office. Consider carefully which rooms will be used by whom and for what. With reference to architecture, "organic" can mean many things. It can refer simply to non-

rectangular form; it can suggest a deeper reverence for the earth (as in the dynamic earthbound designs of Frank Lloyd Wright); it can be a belief that architecture can have a profound effect on our growth and behavior (as in the works of Rudolf Steiner). Then there is the Chinese school of *feng shui*, at the center of which is the notion of designing

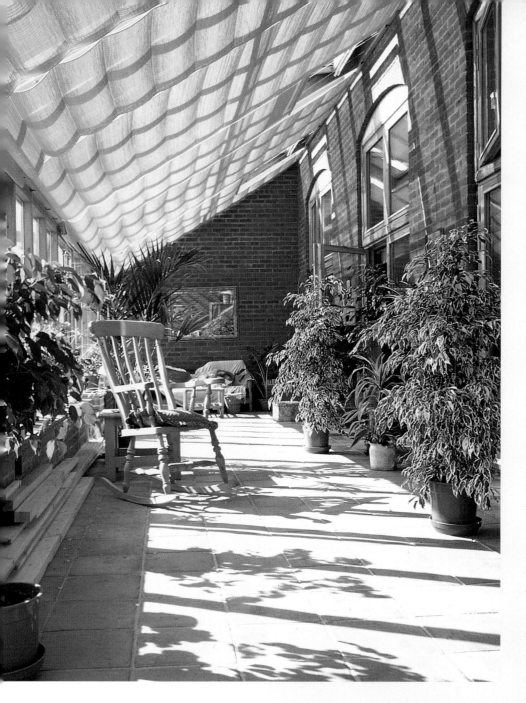

photovoltaic cells), biofuels, wind, and hydro power.

❖ **Optimize** your use of solar energy: a site should be able to see the sun all year-round, so check your winter sun levels, as they are vital to maximizing the solar energy availability. In a city it is best to buy property with a south-facing back garden: there will be less shade and you can add passive and active solar structures – such as a conservatory or solar panels – without too many worries over planning constraints.

❖ **Construct** a garden that requires minimal water, with drought-resistant species and mulches. Collect all rainwater, and use soakaways for any surplus rainwater so that the water table is replenished (especially important in cities where tarmac surfaces are prevalent).

❖ **Hills, other buildings, and trees** can protect a house from prevailing winds or funnel them towards it. Shelter to the west and northeast is generally useful.

❖ **Recycle** nutrients and reduce your water use by using on-site sewage treatment systems. There are many safe and hygienic options, such as compost toilets and reed-bed effluent treatment.

❖ **Minimize and reuse** – minimize refuse from your house by storing and reusing materials and composting on site (*see page 182*). Where possible use local recycling programs.

❖ **Use** as little fossil fuel energy as you can to reach your workplace. If you cannot work from home, travel by public ransportation or bicycle.

surroundings to facilitate the free and healthy flow of *ch'i*, or "life force". Whatever your depth of belief in arts such as *feng shui*, designs incorporating its principles do seem to result in more balanced, peaceful environments.

How healthy is your "organic" space going to be? Lighting, ventilation, and choice of power sources will all have an

BUILDING A SUSTAINABLE HOME

❖ **Plan** the house to use as little fossil fuel as possible. Use materials that did not require huge energy resources to generate or transport, and that will not cause a waste problem or pollution on demolition.

❖ **Aim** to replace fossil fuels with renewable energy from the sun (passive and active solar heating, electricity from

Design for life

effect. A healthy house provides good daylight and sunlight year round, and is well insulated and draft-proof, but well ventilated too. It avoids underground water courses or contaminated soil, and will also minimize the dangers from electromagnetic fields from external sources such as overhead power lines, and internal sources of high voltage, such as television or computer monitors.

insulation

Thermal comfort demands regulation of many factors, from physical activity to humidity, clothing to air temperature and movement. In high humidity the

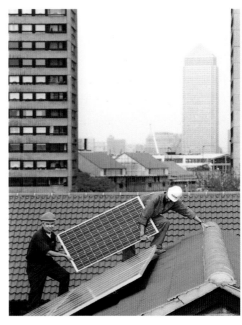

body loses its ability to cool down effectively, and even in warm conditions air movement may be sensed as a cold draft because it increases cooling of the body by convection and evaporation. In the US a large percentage of the drafts that infiltrate houses occur through faulty construction, although a certain amount of ventilation is required in all homes. Make sure all doors and windows are sealed properly and closed tightly against any seals. Check that plaster shrinkage has not left a gap between windows or doors and the adjoining walls; check for gaps between floorboards, skirting boards, and floors, and around pipes and loft hatches. If you can, install a buffer zone between living space and the outside, such as an enclosed porch or greenhouse that acts as an air lock when you venture out.

lighting

We all like a room full of daylight, especially if there is some sunshine, and particularly if the light is coming from more than one direction. Good daylighting can also save energy, since it replaces electric lighting. However, a balance must be found between the saving on electric lighting and heat

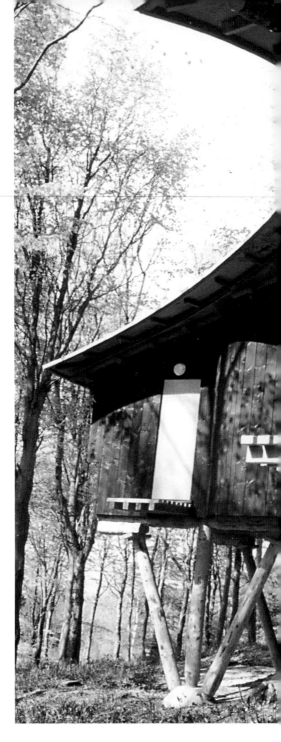

loss from the windows, since they will lose heat at about six times the rate of a wall. Office buildings are good candidates for this kind of energy saving since they are rarely used at night. So how big should a window be? Visit rooms that feel comfortable and imitate

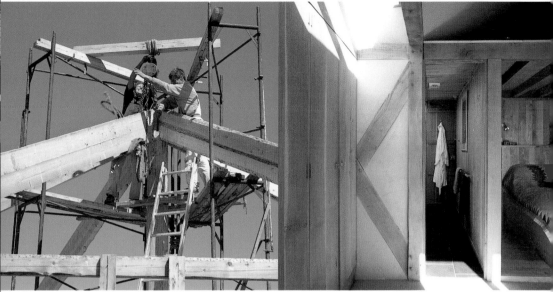

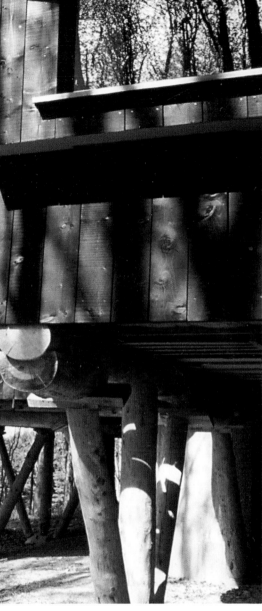

heating

Solar heating is the first choice for heating any space since it is nonpolluting, but on a domestic scale it is rather impractical. Biofuels – waste wood or biogases such as methane – are the next best choice, since their carbon dioxide output is balanced by that taken to grow them sustainably. These are followed by gas, the cleanest fossil fuel, then oil, coal, and finally electricity. Gas and oil boilers will always be able to generate heat faster than those using fuels such as wood and coal. They can run at higher efficiencies without the danger of clogging up with the products of combustion.

electricity

If you have no choice but electricity, you can now opt, in the UK, to buy renewably generated electricity from the "grid". If your offices or company use more than 100 kilowatts per year, you can negotiate to buy your supply from any source you wish. Cheltenham and Gloucester College, for example, buys all its electricity from a local supplier, the Renewable Energy Company. This company generates electricity using methane gas from a waste tip. A large number of domestic users can buy their electricity on a green tariff or from companies such as UnitE.

In the right circumstances you can supply your own power – photovoltaic solar cell arrays are now being integrated into all sorts of buildings, like the offices at the Centre for Alternative Technology in Wales. However, currently the cost of a unit of PV electricity is about ten times that of one bought from the "grid" for the domestic user, and so Britons have some way to go before the PV option is open widely across the UK.

the size and position of the windows and the rooms' proportions and finishes. Windows should be double- or triple-glazed. Where you do need electric light, use the most efficient and long-lasting light bulbs available and only light those rooms that are actually in use.

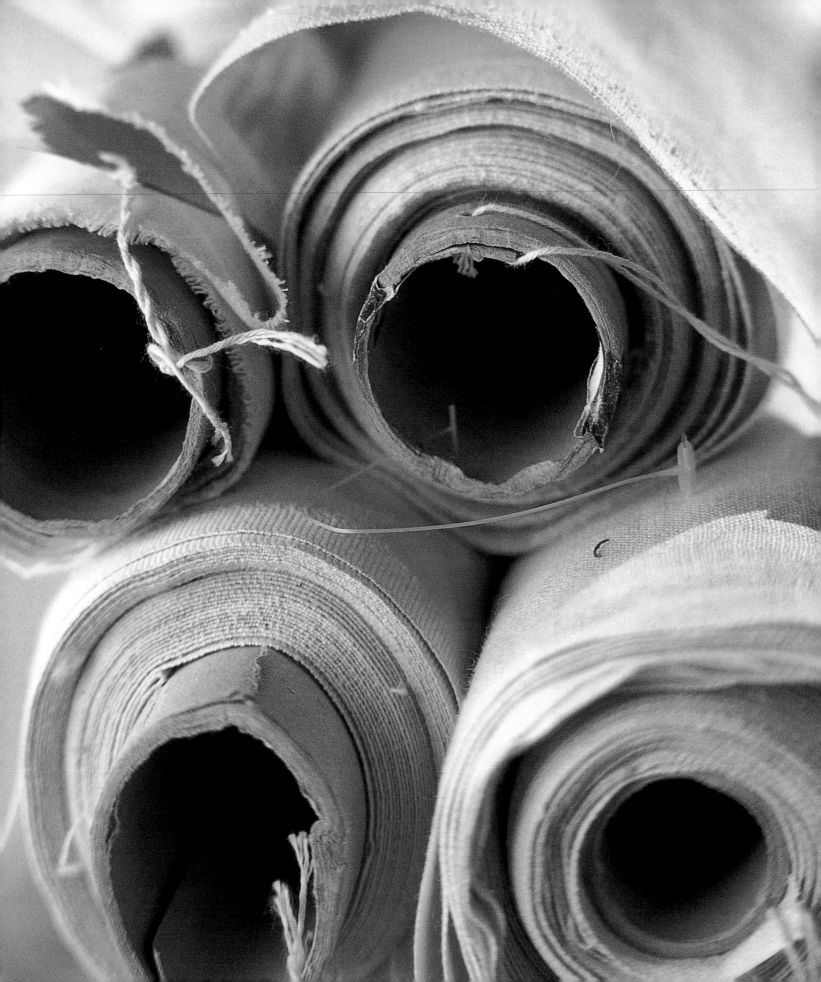

WHY WEAR
organic

Many of us wrestle with "What to wear?", but take a moment to consider the wider implications of the clothes we choose and the impact they may be having on our bodies, on the people who made them and on the planet.

You probably already tend to choose clothes made from natural fibers because they feel good and allow your body to breathe. But did you know that a conventional cotton T-shirt takes ⅓ lb (150 grammes) of pesticides to produce?

SOFTLY DOES IT

The good news is that organic farming and sustainable production methods are not just being applied to the food that we eat, but to other agri-based commodities such as cotton, linen, and wool. While this may be of direct benefit to those who suffer from skin allergies or are chemically sensitive, it is important to all of us who want the products we buy to have been grown and manufactured with environmental consideration.

It is a bonus when you discover that the care that goes into growing the fibers at an agricultural level is supported by extra care and quality control right through the manufacturing process. This results in the softest fabrics imaginable.

Look for natural, pure and nontoxic fabrics in the close-to-the-body-clothes you wear such as underwear, socks, leggings, and T-shirts, or choose organic cotton bed linens and snuggle up to natural comfort. Look, also, for fabrics that, if bleached, dyed, or printed, have used environmentally responsible, low-impact methods such as hydrogen peroxide bleaches and dyes that do not contain heavy metals.

STICK WITH THE NATURAL CHOICES

Try to avoid fabrics with easy care, noniron or crease-resistant finishes. These finishes, which often contain formaldehyde, a known carcinogen, are bonded into the fibers and cannot be washed out. Keep your dry-cleaning to a minimum. The chemicals used in this process are toxic, mainly to the workers at dry-cleaning plants, but there is evidence that we are all exposed to these chemicals when they are released into the environment through air and groundwater pollution.

Wear organic fabrics closest to your skin

Look for pure, nontoxic fabrics

Ask salespeople about how their fabric and clothes are made

Avoid crease-resistant finishes

Keep your dry-cleaning to a minimum

The fabric of society

There is a great range of organic and eco-friendly fabrics available through shops and mail order. From organic cotton underwear to garments made from hemp and recycled fabrics – the choice is yours.

It is now possible to find eco-friendly alternatives to many conventionally produced fabrics. Textiles such as hemp and organic cotton are being increasingly used in clothing and soft furnishings (*see page 186*), and some companies are even developing garments made from recycled fabrics and plastics.

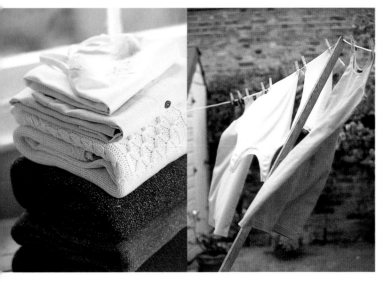

wool

Compared to conventionally grown cotton, conventional wool production uses far fewer chemicals in its manufacturing process. When made into garments, wool is warm in winter, cool in summer, water-resistant on the outside, absorbent on the inside, and naturally flame-resistant. Wool is highly receptive to dyes, so natural, plant-based dyes are a realistic alternative to synthetics in textile production. Wool also naturally repels dirt, thus cutting down on the environmental impact of constant laundering throughout a garment's life.

Because wool is a by-product, it fits well into a sustainable farming system, and because the manufacturing process is relatively uncomplicated, it lends itself to small-scale production and craft-based industry. Look for 100 percent pure new wool garments such as naturally dyed, hand-knitted sweaters, and products such as blankets and throws from small-scale weaving enterprises. Felt-making is another wool-based craft industry that has gained popularity as designers have redefined the craft to produce beautiful felted wool fabrics for hats, shoes, and clothes.

Some people seem to be allergic to wool but, as nearly all conventionally produced wool is routinely moth-proofed with chemicals, it is possible that some of these people are allergic to the moth-proofing rather than the wool.

Unless the woolen products you are buying have been certified as organic in countries such as the Netherlands, Germany, or New Zealand, wool produced in the UK can only be sold as "coming from organic sheep". This means that the wool comes from sheep raised on organic farms, but tells you nothing about the processes the wool has been subjected to after leaving the sheep. This situation is soon to change with the drafting of UK organic textile standards by the Soil Association.

Wool that is organically certified, here in the US, is guaranteed to come from farms where no organophosphate dips have been used on the sheep. Once shorn, the wool is washed without the use of chemicals or bleaches, using soap flakes to remove the lanolin and dirt. It is not chemically treated with moth-proofing or flame-retardant finishes.

Organically certified wool is made into blankets and bedding. It is knitted, often with silk, into fine soft jersey for baby clothes and underwear. Traditionally made, untreated Harris Tweed is made into smart city wear. Sheep skins from organically reared sheep, tanned without the use of harmful chemicals such as chrome, are used to make baby bedding and toys (*see page 125*).

hemp

Hemp is one of the oldest and most versatile plants known to man. It was cultivated for thousands of years throughout the world, primarily as the raw material from which paper, rope, and canvas were made. Due to its strength and weatherproof qualities, hemp was hugely important to the European economy for the manufacture of sails and rigging for sailing ships, and for nets, flags, uniforms, and work clothes.

In the 19th century the mechanization of cotton manufacturing meant that it became possible to produce cotton fabrics more easily and cheaply than hemp, thanks to the labor-intensive processes involved in hemp production. Then jute imported from India began to compete with and replace hemp as the fiber from which ropes and rough industrial fabrics such as sacking were made.

In the 20th century two factors contributed to the almost total obliteration of the hemp industry. The first of these was the banning of hemp-growing, initially in the US in the late 1930s, and then throughout most of the rest of the world, because of its association with marijuana. Although industrial hemp does not

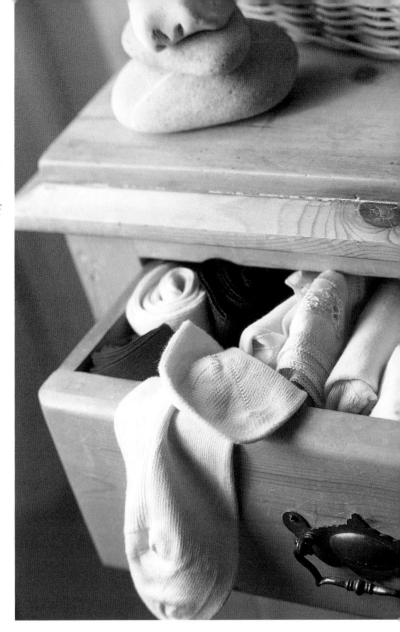

contain sufficient concentrations of tetrahydrocannabinol (THC), the narcotic ingredient in marijuana, to work in the same way as marijuana, the hemp plants were sufficiently similar in appearance to the drug-producing plants to effect a ban. At the same time, the growth in the production of synthetic textiles replaced some of the industrial applications for which hemp's strength had previously had importance, and the industry in Europe

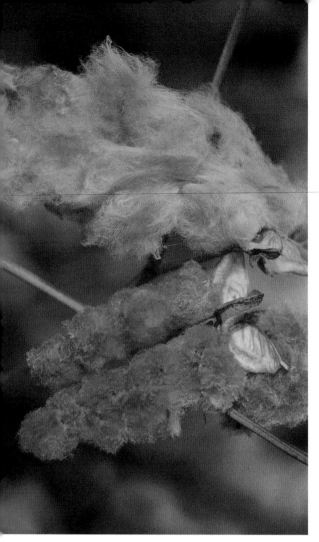

helping to improving soil structure. Hemp also returns a high proportion of nutrients to the soil, as its leaves and roots are left to rot down after harvesting. It is therefore ideal as a rotation crop in a sustainable organic farming system. In fact, farmers have consistently reported higher yields from other crops such as wheat when they have been planted on land after hemp.

Although hemp from China has tested negative for chemical residues, currently there is none that has been certified as organic. Meanwhile Europe, particularly Germany, has enthusiastically re-embraced hemp as an increasingly important eco-fiber and, with the application of modern processing techniques, is producing hemp fabric that is finer and softer than its Chinese counterpart. Some of it is certified organic.

Hemp is used to make beautiful clothes that successfully combine environmental considerations with a radical fashion statement. Similar in appearance to linen, hemp makes stylish shirts, jackets, and suits. Hemp is made into excellent hard-wearing jeans – in fact, Levi Strauss's original jeans were said to be made from hemp and Levi Strauss is now trying to

and America died. That is not the end of the hemp story, however. Hemp cultivation was never banned in China and eastern European countries such as Romania, and these countries are still important sources for hemp fabrics. In the West cultivation of hemp is rapidly rising again as its environmental advantages are increasingly recognized – hemp is now regarded as *the* environmentally friendly fiber.

Hemp is undoubtedly farmed without the use of toxic chemicals, even in China and the former Soviet bloc. It grows without the use of pesticides, and its roots penetrate deep into the soil,

reintroduce the idea. Hemp is also used to make sturdy and practical bags, backpacks, wallets, slippers, canvas shoes, and even sneakers.

cotton

Cotton accounts for nearly half of all the textiles produced in the world today and for a rapidly growing organic industry (*see page 204*). Cotton actually grows in several different colors (*see left*), which can be used to make the ultimate eco-friendly fabrics, since they are created without the need for dyes.

silk

Silk is made from the fine long filaments spun by the silkworm when it makes its cocoon. The silkworm, which is really a caterpillar, is fed entirely on mulberry leaves. The worms are killed when the cocoons are heated in water to release the filaments from the gums that hold it together. Silk is the longest and finest natural textile fiber – with the highest tensile strength – known to man. It is spun and made into lustrous and fine fabrics that are warm in winter, cool in summer and accept dyes more readily than most other fibers. Silk is a huge industry in China. Japan, Thailand, and India also produce silk, although much of the fabric they weave now is made with Chinese yarn. It is hard to ascertain to what extent, if at all, chemicals are used in the farming of mulberry leaves in China. Reputable eco-fabric importers test chinese silk for purity from chemical residues so, if you want to be sure, check that the eco-clothing manufacturer in question sources their silk from one of these importers.

recycled fabrics

The next time you take your old clothes down to your local Salvation Army, do not be embarrassed to include items in a bad condition. If they do not think they will be able to sell them in their shops, they may sell the garment on to recycling merchants. There the garments are sorted by color and fiber content and sold on to mills who specialize in shredding, re-spinning, and weaving, or knitting recycled fabrics. Italy has been home to a thriving recycled wool industry for years and, in the UK, innovative fabrics from all kinds of different fibers – and mixes of fibers – are being developed. Here, in the US an exciting development in recycling technology has enabled polyester fabrics to be made from fibers extruded from recycled plastic bottles (*see right*).

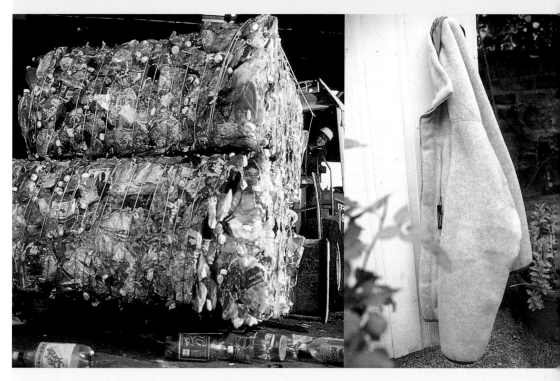

the producers

AN INNOVATIVE APPROACH

Based in Ventura, California, Patagonia make clothing for a variety of activities with an emphasis on durability and innovation. The company cares about the impact of its materials and manufacturing processes on the environment, donating one percent of sales or ten percent of pre-tax profits, whichever is greater, to environmental causes. Patagonia uses organic cotton and hemp, and makes most of its fleece garments from post-consumer recycled (PCR®) plastic (*see above left*), which brings significant environmental savings and advantages. Most of its dyes are low-impact; many fabric finishes are free of formaldehyde and chlorine. The company's stores and facilities also incorporate a variety of eco-friendly building techniques.

To us, quality means more than how a garment looks or functions; it also includes the way it affects the environment.

YVON CHOUINARD, FOUNDER, PATAGONIA CLOTHING COMPANY

Focus on cotton

Naturally kinder for you and for the environment, the growing range of organically certified cotton fabrics offers you the natural choice next to your skin and is helping to improve standards of living for others.

One of the world's most widely traded commodities, cotton accounts for roughly half of all the textiles produced worldwide. Although cotton has been successfully promoted as "pure" and "natural", the modern production and processing of conventional cotton is far from natural.

natural fibers

Conventionally farmed cotton is one of the world's most intensively produced crops, treated with a barrage of chemicals, including fertilizers, pesticides, growth regulators, and defoliants. In response to growing environmental, economic, and social concerns, both in the developed and the developing world, many cotton farmers and manufacturers have converted to sustainable production methods. Organic cotton was first grown in the late 1980s by a cooperative in Turkey that wanted to demonstrate that sustainable farming methods need not be limited to food production. The cultivation of organic cotton soon spread to the US, where some conventional growers were starting to worry about the rapid escalation of pesticide use, and to Peru, where organic cotton was seen as a radical solution for subsistance farmers for whom coca had previously been the only cash crop (*see page 104*). Egypt has become another primary producer of organic cotton, with projects such as the Sekem biodynamic initiative (*see below left*) growing organically and supporting communities. As demand easily outstrips supply, cultivation of organic cotton is increasing worldwide.

cotton traders

Because the cotton production chain from grower to consumer is complex, and environmental hazards occur throughout its length, organic textile standards have been developed to govern the use of chemicals on the farm and throughout the manufacturing process. Thus consumers can be sure that the cotton in the organically certified products they buy was not only grown using sustainable farming methods, but bleached without the use of chlorine bleaches and dyed without the use of environmentally damaging toxic dyes.

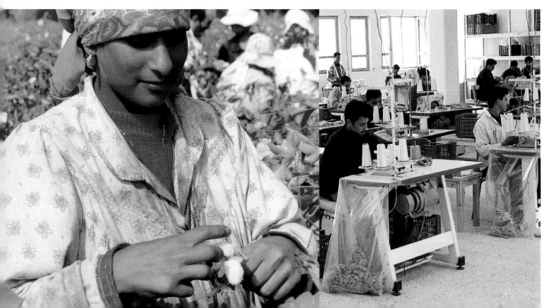

THE DIFFERENCES THAT COUNT

❖ It is estimated that conventional cotton accounts for nearly 25 percent of the total global insecticide market: organic farming methods do not place farm workers at risk of exposure to toxic chemicals, and do not reduce soil fertility or pollute groundwater

❖ Organic cotton is not genetically modified: GM cotton has been grown here in the US since 1996

❖ Farmers in the developing world grow organic cotton in rotation with food crops, enabling them to feed their families and animals at the same time as producing a valuable cash crop for export

❖ Fabrics made from organic cotton are not colored using heavy metal dyes, bleached with chlorine bleaches, or treated with formaldehyde

❖ Organic cotton is kinder to you and to the environment: by choosing it, consumers are supporting sustainable practices and processing methods, and helping to secure better conditions for plantation workers

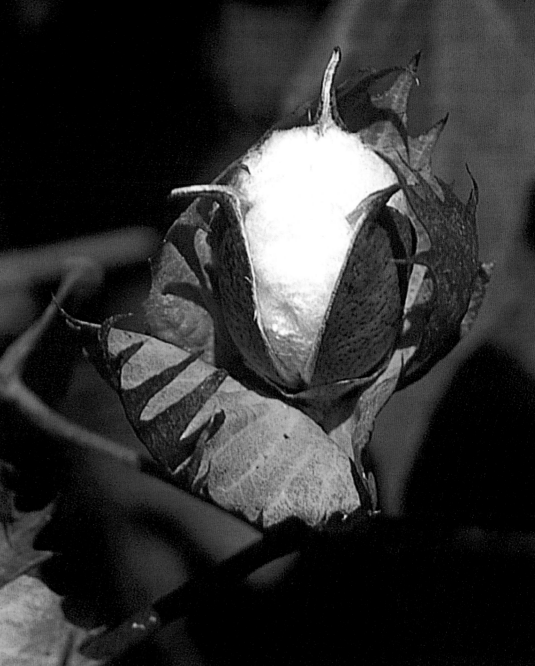

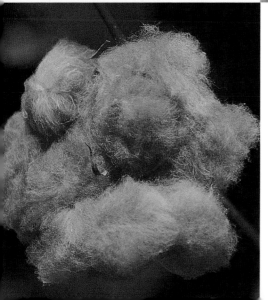

Some producers grow colored cotton, eliminating the need for dyes altogether (*see page 202*). Organic cotton is often knitted into jersey fabrics, since this avoids some of the environmental impact associated with the use and subsequent removal of yarn strengtheners in the weaving process. Many of the clothes that are available – made from soft, stretchy organic cotton jersey – are the garments we wear next to our skin: underwear, socks, and T-shirts. Some companies, such as Patagonia (*see page 203*), are committed to using only organic cotton in their garments. Other manufacturers, such as Levi, Gap, and Nike, are blend organic cotton with conventional cotton to support the organic cotton market.

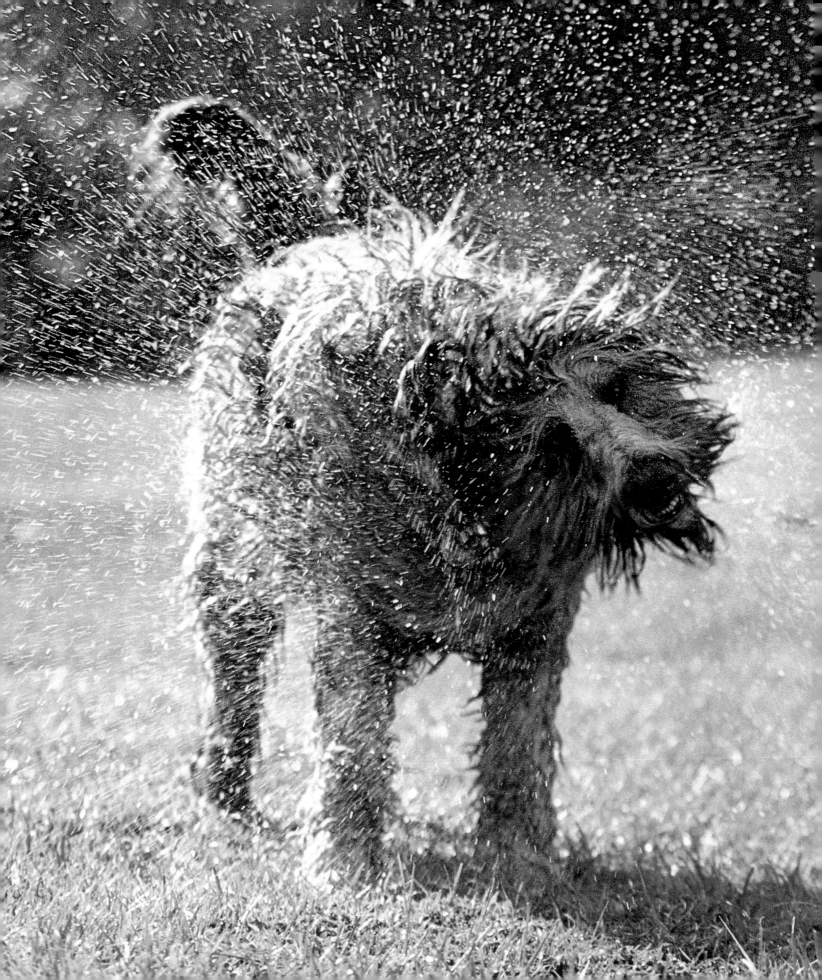

WHY GO organic

With so many American households owning at least one pet, they are a key part of our lives. Our pets bring us great joy, and caring for them is important.

Owning a pet is a great responsibility, but brings great rewards. Just as you care for your children, it is up to you to feed and care for your pet, and to provide it with a safe, stimulating environment. How you choose to nurture your pet has a major effect on its health and happiness, so it is good to know that many of the choices you make for yourself and your family you can make for your pets too. The choices are easy to make, and there is plenty of information to help you (*see page 223*).

FEEDING YOUR PETS

When we start to question the effects of artificial substances in our own food, it is only natural to consider what goes into the foods we give our pets. Most owners who routinely feed their animals cans and packages of processed pet foods might be surprised to learn that these are permitted to contain over 100 chemical additives. It may be less of a surprise to know that our pets are, in fact, just as susceptible as we are to the effects of any pesticides, fertilizers, and additives used in food production. Happily, it is as easy to convert our pets' diets to organic as it is our own, and most domestic pets can be fed on the same organic foods, including fruit, vegetables, and meats, that we might choose for ourselves. There is, however, a growing number of organic processed pet foods coming on to the market, particularly for dogs and cats, giving you the convenient option when circumstances dictate.

YOUR PET'S HEALTH & ENVIRONMENT

A balanced organic diet should ensure your pet's good health. When illnesses do occur, however, there are plenty of alternatives to conventional treatments to consider. Herbalism, homeopathy, and aromatherapy are as effective on animals as on humans, although it is always wise to seek specific veterinary advice. There are also natural alternatives and guidelines to consider when looking after your pets and giving them a healthy, happy environment.

Feed your pets a balanced diet of fresh organic foods where possible, according to species-specific requirements

Seek out natural healthcare alternatives to conventional treatments for pets

Create a safe and healthy environment for your pet to enjoy

Control dog fleas with an essential oils spray or a herb-packed collar

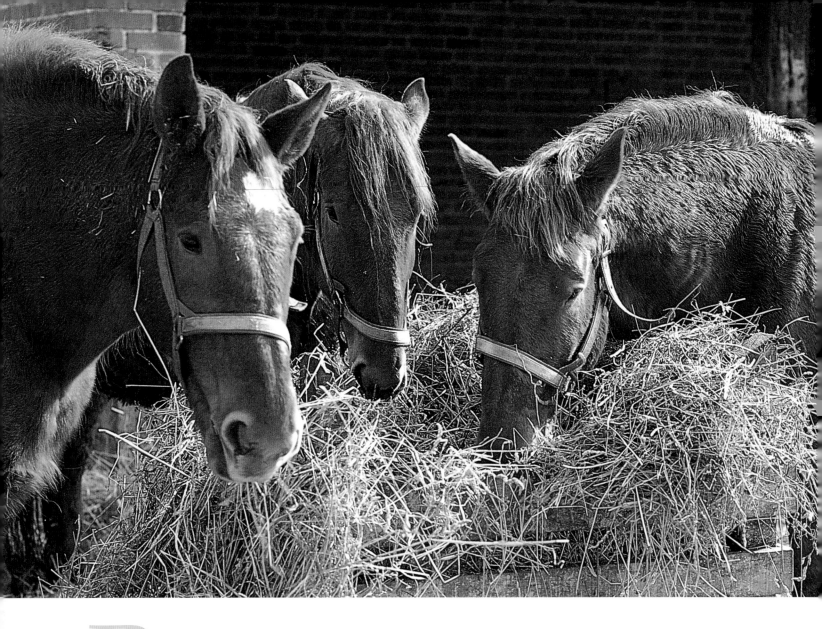

Pet subjects

Our pets and animals are dependent upon us for almost all of their needs, so how we feed and nourish them and how we care for them will have a strong influence on their health and happiness.

What we feed our pets and animals is probably the single most important factor in their health and well-being. General rules are that fresh food is always best, variety is important and compatibility with an animal's species-specific needs is vital. Some countries have organzations that provide common-sense principles concerning your pet's nutrition and health. The British Association of Holistic Nutrition and Medicine (BAHNM), for example, has a holistic symbol program, through which the symbol is awarded to products whose full ingredients have been certified compatible with the target species. The BAHNM is also able to advise on using other noncertified foods and products. However, freedom from the traces of artificial chemicals found in conventional foods should also be a key consideration and, as in humans, this is where organically produced foods play a key role. For authentication of organic pet food and supplements, the Soil Association and Demeter symbols are the ones to look out for in the UK. But there are many others, worldwide, that are approved by the Soil Association. Different symbols require different levels of stringency in what is meant by "organic", although these parameters are regularly updated.

The threat of genetically modified organisms (GMOs) is present for animal foods as it is for human foods, so choosing organic is the best way to fight this threat and say NO to GMOs.

feeding dogs

Although the commercial pet food industry has thrived by producing food to a theoretically adequate formula of basic nutrients, a diet of solely canned or bagged dry food is no more enjoyable or nutritionally desirable for your dog than it would be for you. Like many processed foods, the average dog foods often contain many of the artificial flavorings and chemical additives that we should all try to avoid. By and large, giving a dog a lot of what we eat ourselves is the soundest way to good nutrition, with organic alternatives being the most healthy option. This means feeding your dog a balanced diet that includes fruit and vegetables. These are musts for dogs, as only around a third of their diet should be made up of meat. A variety of forms and types of fruit and vegetables is valuable, from raw chunky to raw grated and even lightly cooked vegetables. Add organic herbs such as freshly chopped garlic, watercress, parsley, and powdered kelp and you have a really tasty and well-formulated diet. In addition, dogs should have, if possible, raw organic bones and pieces of raw organic meat for chewing on, and raw "green" tripe. As the demand for organic food continues to rise, organic canned and dried pet foods are becoming more available in some specialty stores. They are not advisable for full-

PET FOOD PLATTERS

It is best to use ceramic, clay, stoneware, or enamel feeding receptacles for your pet. Food bowls made of plastic are not a good idea, since the chemical itself and the dense dyeing matter usually used to color it can leach into food and water quite easily. The toxic effects of such materials are well-proven, and many dogs have benefited from disposal of their plastic bowls.

SOURCING & STORING FOOD

Since it is always best to feed your pets fresh, unprocessed foods when you can, it is probably wise not to indulge in the habit of bulk-buying if you can avoid it. Suitable foods can be deep-frozen, such as raw meat – organic if possible. Food containers should be rat-proof and not prone to condensation. Dried organic foods, such as dog biscuits, should be stored in a cool, dark and dry place.

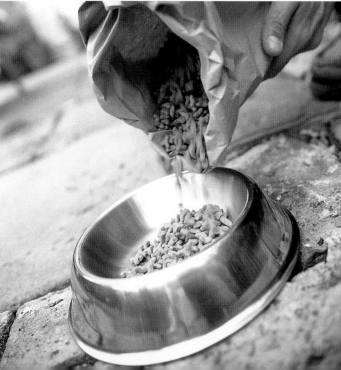

Pet subjects

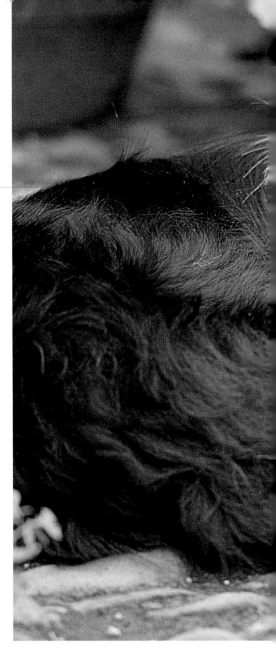

time use but for occasional feedings they are preferable to nonorganic products. It is also a good idea to prepare your own organic treats or offer slices of raw organic carrot or squares of organic bread or toast.

feeding cats

Although the same basic principles for feeding dogs apply to cats, they do have some special considerations. Unlike dogs, cats are dependent on some meat or fish in their diet, due to the essential amino acids these contain. Cats struggle to tolerate some vegetables, such as the onion family, including garlic. Cats' oral and dental health is just as dependent on meat and bones to chew as dogs', but they are very susceptible to salmonella food poisoning. Foods must be fresh, therefore, and careful hygiene in preparation is vital. Organic canned and dried cat foods are available for occasional use. Look out for a wide range of organic cat food on the internet.

feeding birds

Domestic caged birds are necessarily even more dependent upon us than uncaged animals. Each species has different nutritional requirements. If possible, buy organic seeds for your birds and organic fresh fruit particular to each species' natural home.

feeding rabbits & rodents

As with all pets, rabbits, and small rodents should be given fresh, wholesome food, preferably organic. Rabbits will survive very well on grass and other herbage, as well as on fresh vegetables. Hay is a good form of food and bedding but it must not be moldy. Hay should be organic, but if not, it should at least come from ground that has not been treated with artificial fertilizers. Organic hay is also good for most small rodents but some of these, especially chinchillas, are more adapted than rabbits to eating fresh fruit. In the absence of organic fresh fruit, organic dried fruits are a good alternative. There are organic preprepared foods you can use, but preferably only occasionally.

feeding horses

The dietary considerations for horses are more complex than for dogs and cats.

All the same principles apply, however: foods should be fresh, varied, compatible with the species, and, when possible, organically produced. Feeding your horse grains is not desirable, unless you are making up for the energy requirements of very strenuous work schedules. Hay should be from organic land if possible, or at least from ground that has not been treated with artificial fertilizers. The horse is a strictly herbivorous species and

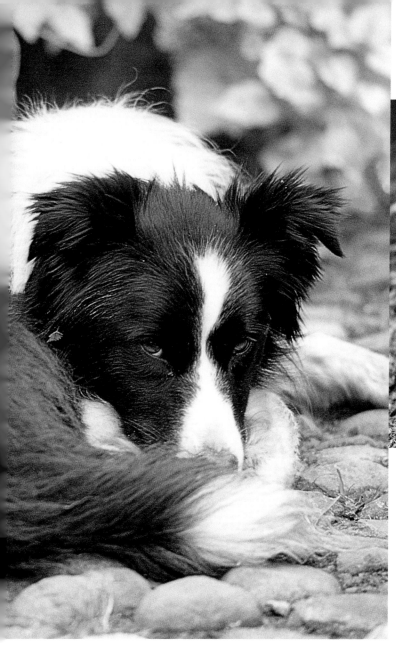

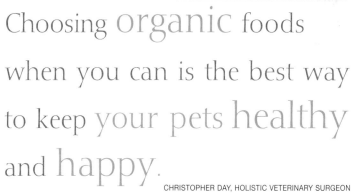

Choosing organic foods when you can is the best way to keep your pets healthy and happy.

CHRISTOPHER DAY, HOLISTIC VETERINARY SURGEON

horses should never be fed foods and supplements containing animal products. It is best, too, to avoid molasses and other sugary materials, including sugar beet. Most of the commercially produced foods currently available fall short of these common-sense requirements. Accurate and careful reading of the bags will tell the full story, and it is advisable to read labels in detail. Chaffs are usually coated in molasses, even if you do not expect

them to be. Most compound feeds contain molasses, and some contain animal products. Some feeds contain preservatives and other artificial additives to accommodate milling and storage. The best diet for a horse is organic grass or hay, or at least grass or hay from ground that has not been treated with artificial fertilizers. If this needs supplementing, herbs should be selected to source extra vitamins and minerals. If

grain is required, oats and bran can be used, provided that adequate calcium rebalancing is practiced, for example by the addition of ground limestone or limestone flour. Barley can be offered if the horse needs to gain weight, and boiled linseed or cooked linseed cake is a useful energy, protein, and oil supplement. Be wary of the many herbal supplements now available for horses. This is a lucrative market, because people

Pet subjects

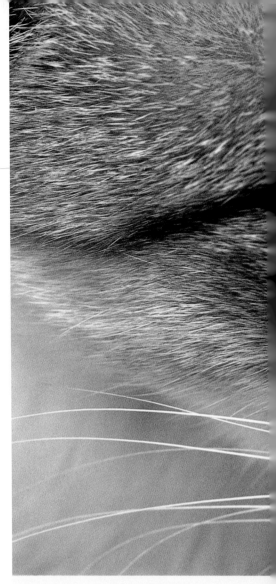

want to do the best for their horses, but the marketing can be misleading. Some have names or labels that imply medical benefits that have not been substantiated.

pet health

The area of pet health care products is one that many pet owners find very confusing. Although advice abounds, it can often seem conflicting and may be offered out of a vested interest. If your animal appears healthy, and if he or she is on a wholesome, preferably organic, diet, then nutritional or health supplements should not be necessary. If the animal is not healthy, you should seek the advice of a veterinarian who is well versed or preferably qualified in the specialist areas of natural medicine, nutrition, and holistic thinking. Although, as is the case for humans, conventional medicines are useful for treating some diseases, for others "alternative" treatments can offer a more natural option. Homeopathic medicines are available over-the-counter for most first-aid indications, and Bach's Rescue Remedy can be of invaluable support for conditions of sudden onset, such as shock, fright or panic. Herbs such as skullcap and valerian or the

application of lavender oil can help in times of anticipated stress, but always seek veterinary advice first.

supplements

There are some occasions when supplements, including vitamins and herbs, may be advised. Vitamin B may relieve stress and Vitamin C may help connective tissues and the immune system. Herbal echinacea can support the immune system in times of challenge, and garlic is good for deterring worms, and as a disinfectant, insect repellent, and immune stimulant. In the case of blood-related conditions, such as anemia, an integrated homeopathic and nutritional approach is required rather than some off-the-shelf concoction. If pasture land or hay for horses is not of high quality, then a formula of herbs should be put together for your horse, depending on its special needs. If such things as hoof formation go wrong, again an integrated homeopathic and nutritional program is needed. In cases of arthritis in dogs, cats, and horses, natural medicines can be used, but there is also a range of magnetic devices available, although it is not very easy to tell in advance which patients will be helped and which ones will not.

SQUEAKY CLEAN

Although shampooing animals is mostly unnecessary, natural-based shampoos are available and are often based on essential oils such as tea tree. Be sure to avoid products made by companies who perform animal experiments and tests. If an actual medication is required for the skin, coal tar, and sulphur shampoos can prove very useful, but are not particularly environmentally sensitive. Routine shampooing of any animal can prove damaging to its coat and skin. Problems with fleas can usually be controlled

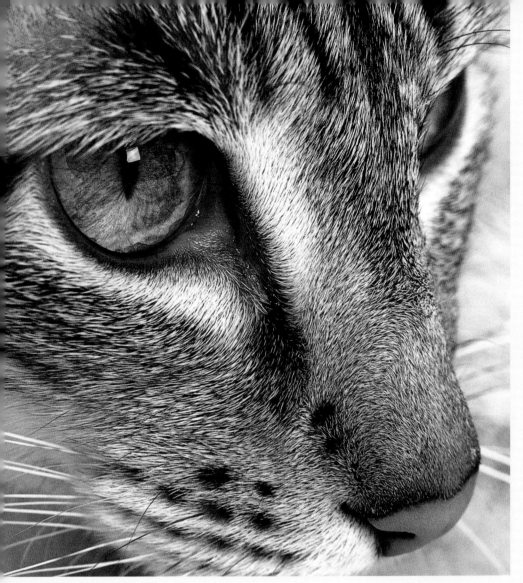

breed and size, but you should be careful not to play too hard when the weather is hot.

Caged birds should have as large a cage as possible and the freedom of a room or large aviary should be a daily allowance. Humidity, temperature, and drafts must be controlled as much as possible. Access to unfiltered sunlight is also very valuable but beware overheating. Suitable perches should be provided and positioned far enough from the floor or ground to prevent soiling of tail feathers. Food and fresh, clean water should be available for 24 hours a day.

For rabbits and small rodents, special considerations are bedding, which should preferably be organic hay, and toys, which should be hazard-free. For instance, ensure that nothing is put in the cage which could entangle the animal.

Horses are a special case. They need space, companions, grazing facilities, shade, a field shelter for their use in inclement weather, a roomy and well-bedded, well-ventilated, draft-free stable, and fresh water. Straw seems to be the most comfortable bedding material of all, as long as it is both plentiful and clean. Organic is best, especially for horses who eat their bedding. Rugging in wintertime is essential for clipped horses, even in a stable, but usually not for horses with a good winter coat, even if kept outside. As mentioned before, a good field shelter is advisable, especially since long periods of rain and wind can be very chilling.

without the use of the toxic pesticides present in commercial sprays and powders. Adding yeast or garlic to your animal's food or cider vinegar to its water will make your pet less tasty to fleas. Alternatively, make up water sprays containing citrus essential oils with which to spray your pet, or pack pennyroyal mint into a fabric collar that it can wear.

PET TERRITORIES

It is vital for the welfare of your animal that he or she should have a suitable environment in which to live. Both dogs and cats require some private area, where they can be out of harm's way and safe from family feet when they choose. In most cases, pets enjoy human company and the bedding area should be near the family. Cats often like an elevated position that they can call their own. Dogs should be provided with a bed that is not in a draft or on a damp floor. Watch out for the heating effect of pipes along skirting boards or under floors nearby and try to avoid see-sawing temperatures in wintertime. Dogs must be given plenty of exercise, according to

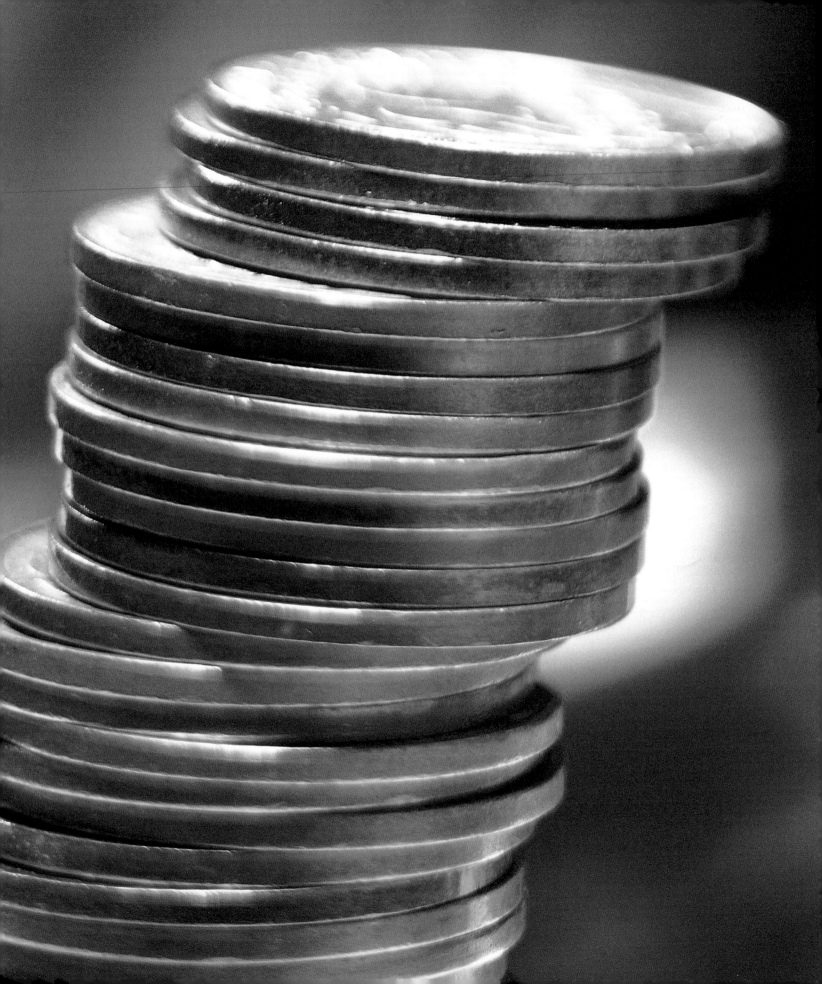

WHY ORGANIC finance

Investing in eco-ethical finance is the feel-good, positive way to make your money work for you and what you believe in. It is the win-win, caring, sharing, street-wise form of finance.

The concept of eco-ethical finance first began in the 1970s and has now blossomed into the fastest-growing sector of the money market. In the UK, where eco-finance is booming, eco-ethical investments exploded to £2.5 billion in the 1990s and are expected to triple by 2005.

A PROFITABLE PARTNERSHIP

Eco-ethical finance has nothing to hide and conducts its business in a totally transparent way. Eco-ethical finance places business, social, ethical, and environmental needs in genuine partnership. Unlike conventional alternatives, eco-ethical finance benefits everyone and everything – especially the environment – and it is this qualitative difference that makes it unique. Though both systems use mostly the same investment vehicles, conventional finance only looks at financial return and security. Eco-ethical finance looks at the social and environmental effects as well.

Eco-ethical finance works in exactly the same way as conventional finance. It offers just as many options, the rates are just as competitive, and the quality of service and level of advice and expertise are often better. Research shows that the track records of eco-finance investments match those of their nonethical counterparts, thus proving that finance with a heart can make you money too.

SHARED IDEALS

As with organic food and farming, and fair trade, eco-ethical finance offers people a sense of personal involvement and shared ideals. And because different people feel strongly about different issues, eco-ethical finance allows you to tailor your investments to suit your personal ethical or environmental portfolio. It is, in short, the finance for today's caring consumers who want to invest in the future. It could be the most positive and rewarding step of your life.

Open an account with a "green" bank

Buy fairly traded goods where possible

Invest in eco-ethical finance – the positive way to make money work for you

Tailor your investments to suit your ethical portfolio

Making your money count

One in three consumers is already using purse power to bring about worldwide environmental and social improvements, helping to create a better world for everyone.

WHERE TO START WITH YOUR ECO-PORTFOLIO

Seek advice

Ask for brochures

Read up as much as you can

Check out a company's eco-credibility if you are thinking of using them: do they deal only with eco-ethical businesses, or with conventional financial institutions as well?

Ask for a company's list of eco- and ethical criteria before dealing with them

Check whether a company you are thinking of using, or are already using, operates positive or negative financing

Saving and investing your money in eco-ethical programs, and choosing to spend it on organic, eco-friendly and ethically sound goods is a simple way to help the market to grow and flourish – over five million workers, for example, are supported by fair trade programs, and organic food is the fastest-growing sector of the food market in many countries. "Green" tourism is another development that is having a major impact, since tourism is the world's biggest industry.

INVESTING IN A BETTER WORLD

Saving with ethical finance companies who invest positively also has a direct effect on what happens in the future. Investing your money in pension funds with socially responsible criteria has an added effect and puts pressure on companies with negative criteria to make changes.

More than 400,000 people now use credit unions. These enable people living or working in the same place to save and borrow at affordable rates. Micro-finance has helped millions of people and businesses to find their feet. In the UK, the largest, The Prince's Trust, has helped 35,000 young people between the ages of 18 and 30 start over 30,000 businesses. In Bangladesh the Grameen Bank, founded by an economics professor, Mohammed Yunus, in the 1970s, has helped millions to escape from poverty. It makes loans to people – mainly women – with less than half an acre of land.

Also gaining official recognition are alternative currencies, based on people's worth and skills. "Time Banks" and "Time Money" programs, such as Fair Shares or Time Dollar here in the US, allow you to use your time as money. Local currencies for local people operate at village level and in cyberspace on the internet, while another program, the Local Exchange Trading System (LETS), is a European skill-swapping currency that enables people to earn credit by trading their skills.

ECO-ETHICAL BANKS

Socially responsible banks offer a full range of services and various saving options. They approach "green" finance in two broad ways:

Negative – banks that avoid financing or investing in companies and projects that have a negative impact on the environment and the community.

Positive – banks that only finance or invest in companies and projects that have a positive impact on the environment and the community. Triodos Bank (*see below*) invests only in ventures that are ecologically and socially sustainable as well as financially sound. The only main street bank to cater seriously to the eco-ethical investor is the Co-operative Bank. Its policy is determined in consultation with customers. Its Customers Who Care program campaigns on various issues and has raised funds for several organizations. It also has an internet banking service, Smile.

"ECO" CREDIT CARDS

These offer everyday shoppers an easy, simple way to support an organization that you believe in every time you shop. Hundreds exist, including those

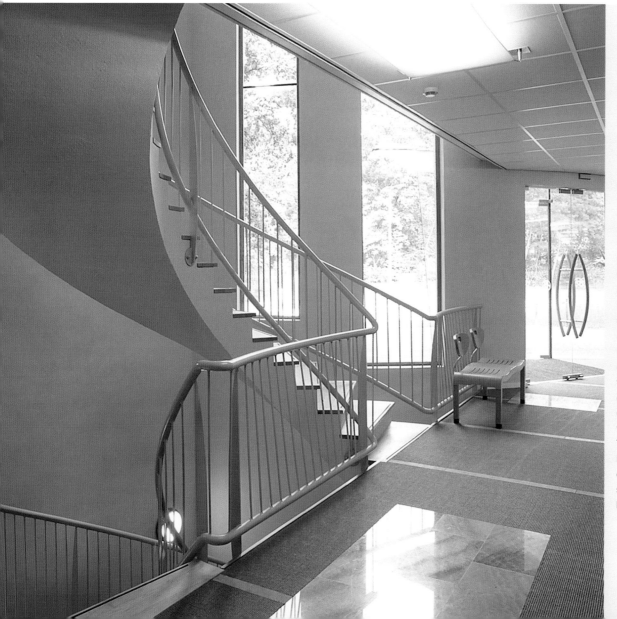

TRIODOS BANK

Founded in 1980, Triodos Bank has offices in the Netherlands, the UK, and Belgium. Organic food and farming, renewable energy, social housing, fair trade, and micro-credit are given high priorities. Its partnership savings accounts include the Organic Saver and Earth Saver. Triodos Match is a green business angels "matching service", bringing green investors together with like-minded entrepreneurs who are looking for finance for their businesses. The bank publishes regular newsletters and a complete list of projects financed. Its new Dutch eco-office in Utrechtseweg (*see left*) fits in perfectly with its green surroundings. The design was influenced by the bank's aim of constructing the most sustainable, low-energy building possible.

Making your money count

STEP-BY-STEP GUIDE TO ECO-FINANCE

Where your money goes:

✤ Organic farming

✤ Energy conservation, e.g. solar energy

✤ Conservation

✤ Sustainable housing

✤ "Green" transportation

✤ Community welfare; equal pay and equal rights; fair trade

✤ Positive healthcare

✤ Animal welfare

✤ Social, environmental businesses; charities

Where your money does not go:

✤ Intensive farming; genetically modified organisms (GMOs)

✤ Nuclear energy

✤ Production of chloro-fluorocarbons (CFCs) and ozone-depleting chemicals (ODCs); pesticides; deforestation; water pollution

✤ Exploitation of the developing world; unfair employment policies

✤ Testing on animals

✤ Tobacco

✤ Environmentally damaging businesses

✤ Armaments, human rights abuse, pornography

issued by HDRA – the organic organization, Oxfam, and the Centre for Alternative Technology. The Co-operative Bank's Greenpeace Affinity card is the only biodegradable one on the market.

ECOLOGY BUILDING SOCIETY

The Ecology Building Society, in the UK, was founded in 1981 to improve the environment by promoting sustainable housing and communities. It offers savings accounts and specializes in mortgages on properties and small-scale ventures that give an ecological payback. Supporting it enables more organic farmers and ecological businesses to thrive. Investors receive regular newsletters. Recent projects include renovation of a traditional watermill in Frome, England.

ETHICS WITH PROFITS

There are many different ways to invest ethically. "Green" pension funds enable you to save for your old age without sacrificing your principles. There are currently over 40 different funds, of varying shades of green and with different socially responsible portfolios. Seek advice from independent eco-ethical financial advisers, who offer advice on the full range of eco-ethical options available, and keep abreast of ethical financial institutions and green pension funds to see how far they match their ideals.

One such example is the Ethical Investors Group, which was established in 1989 to provide independent, socially responsible advice. Like Triodos Bank (*see page 217*), it deals exclusively in positive investment. Uniquely, 50 percent of net business profits are distributed to organizations nominated by clients, which means investing through it also allows you to support your favorite eco-organization. Another example is the Ethical Investment Co-operative Ltd, in the UK, which is a cooperative positive investment group that predominantly services the north of the country.

"GREEN" INSURANCE

Companies around the globe such as Naturesave Policies and Animal Friends Insurance Services are part of a developing industry that aims to encourage environmentally aware insurance and trading policies. Naturesave offers home and travel insurances, and allocates 10 percent of premiums to its trust to fund environmental and conservation projects. Animal Friends Insurance Services is a nonprofit insurance service that does not necessarily invest positively, but its profits go to animal welfare causes.

SHARING THE LOAD

Similar to a building society, Shared Interest is a form of cooperative lending society, established in 1990 in England, that enables savers to form fair trade savings partnerships with people working in the developing world. Savers lend part of their savings to workers to enable them to earn a better living in return for a fair return.

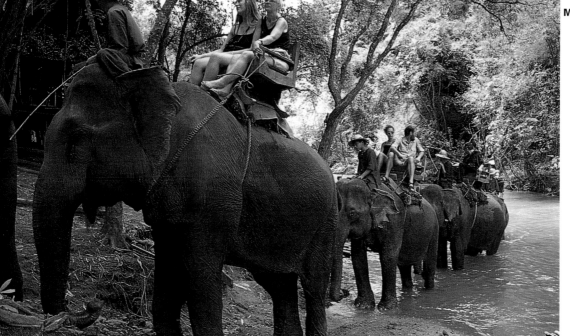

COMMUNITY CAPITAL

Many micro-finance programs are working worldwide at local level. These enable people who are unable to get finance from conventional banks to start up. A British company, ICOF Community Capital, for example, offers people the chance to invest in their own and other local communities.

EXERCISING YOUR CHOICE

Organic consumerism is about taking charge of your own money, both spending it and saving it, in ways that matter to you. Whether you want to support organic farming by buying organic food, do your bit for the environment by choosing eco-friendly products, buy fair trade goods to help support the developing world, or ensure your money is not invested in armaments, that choice is now possible. For the first time in recent economic history, as various consumer campaigns have shown, consumers are discovering that we can have more influence in this way than in any other. One in

three consumers are already using their purse power to make things change for the collective better. As a result, consumers around the world are creating a new kind of caring economy for themselves. This in turn is having a significant influence on conventional economic models and the way other companies do their business.

GREEN TOURISM

The "greening" of the world's largest industry – tourism – is an important, exciting development. Vacations in the sun and travel to exotic destinations are the stuff of which dreams are made. But while we have a wonderful time, tourism brings problems. In developing countries the impact of tourism can change the way of life irrevocably, yet local people do not necessarily benefit and often pay the greatest price in terms of social, cultural, and environmental costs. Green tourism is a means of providing nonexploitative holidays. Your green dreams start here.

The green tourist

"There came a point at which I started to question why the travel industry, now the biggest industry in the world, was failing so miserably in its ability to create and spread wealth, help eliminate poverty, generate jobs, and secure the futures of important wilderness areas, particularly in developing countries. Too often the real cost of one's holiday is wrapped in the intangible but very high social, environmental, and cultural cost borne by one's hosts … Today there is a choice as to how and where you spend your holiday money. Pioneering new initiatives, community projects, eco-tourism companies, organizations, and visionaries are leading the way in 'greening' travel and saving cultures and wilderness areas for future generations to enjoy and respect too."

JULIAN MATTHEWS,
FOUNDER AND DIRECTOR,
DISCOVERY INITIATIVES

It's a fair crop

As the term suggests, fair trade initiatives have led producers in all parts of the developing world to enjoy a fairer return for their skills, by providing better working conditions and an improved standard of living.

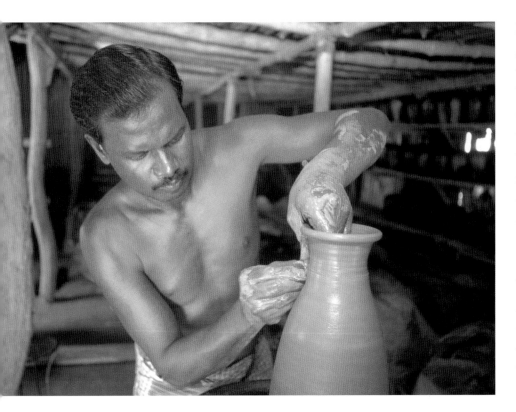

Buying organic and fairly traded food, and other goods that have been produced and sold according to socially and environmentally responsible criteria, brings many rewards. This positive form of trading offers security (suitable working conditions and fair wages) and improved quality of life for workers in the developing world, as well as a clean conscience for consumers and a better environment. The aims of fair trade and organic farming complement each other very well, and more products are being developed that are both organic and fairly traded.

WHAT FAIR TRADE MEANS

As Phil Wells, Director of the Fairtrade Foundation, explains, "Fair trade organizations are companies – often owned by charities such as Oxfam and Traidcraft – that buy and sell products from poor or disadvantaged producers in the developing world

From this work I earn money and can live happily with my

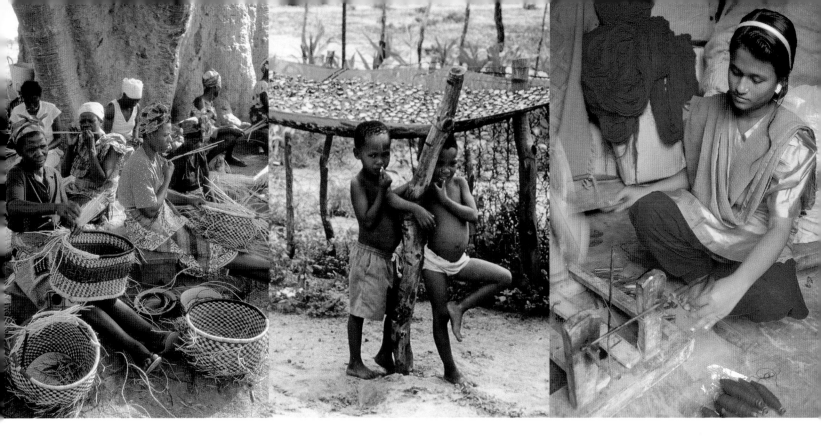

in order to enable them to have more secure lives." Products are sold through stores, mail order, or a network of volunteers and include handcrafted items, clothing, and food products. The producers benefit from on-going trading so they can plan for their future, have democratic rights and decide for themselves how profits should be utilized.

In recent years fairly traded products have begun to appear in supermarkets, denoted by the Fairtrade Mark. The Fairtrade Mark can be found on coffees, teas, chocolate, cocoa, orange juice, bananas, and honey. The Fairtade Mark guarantees consumers that these goods are genuinely fairly traded. Fairtrade labeling organizations now exist in 18 countries and all use the same international standards. Oxfam also has a FairTrade symbol for goods produced under its fair trade programs.

HELPING PEOPLE TO HELP THEMSELVES

For people producing fairly traded items in the developing world the benefits are clear. Ram Chandra Patel (*left*), a potter based in the village of Kakran, Bangladesh, gets better work and wages producing items for the Oxfam FairTrade range. For Agana Ageya, part of the Bolgatanga Basket Weavers' Club Cooperative in Ghana (*above left*), supplying Oxfam with woven baskets is essential: "It means that families can have enough to eat, we can pay for our children's schooling, and we can buy medicines if someone is ill." Asiya Akter (*above right*), one of a group of weavers based near Dhaka, Bangladesh, remarks: "We are earning more than others outside the group and getting regular payment." Other fairly traded projects, such as the Herbs in Africa initiative (*see above center and page 63*) are reaping similar rewards.

Encouragement & expansion

"Fairtrade labeling on foods is encouraging commercial companies to develop foods on a similar basis, so that consumers can get fairly traded foods in supermarkets too. In this way, far more fairtrade products can be sold, and more producers benefit."

PHIL WELLS, DIRECTOR,
FAIRTRADE FOUNDATION

whole family. FairTrade means better work and more orders.

RAM CHANDRA PATEL, POTTER, KAKRAN, BANGLADESH

The Organic Directory

Who to contact

The following are addresses for organizations you may wish to contact for further information.
E-mail and/or website addresses are in **bold**.

organic organizations

ORGANIC TRADE ASSOCIATION

PO Box 547
Greenfield, MA 01302
413-774-7511
f: 413-774-6432

www.ota.com

ORGANIC MATERIALS REVIEW INSTITUTE

PO Box 11558
Eugene, OR 97440
541-343-7600
f: 541-343-8971

www.omri.org
OMRI is a nonprofit organization that provides a newsletter and profess-ional, independent, and transparent review of materials and compatible processes allowed to produce, process, and handle organic food and fiber.

COMMUNITY ALLIANCE WITH FAMILY FARMERS (CAFF)

P.O. Box 363
Davis, CA 95617
Phone: 530 756-8518
fax: 530 756-7857
web site: www.caff.org
e-mail: nod@caff.org

ORGANIC CONSUMERS ASSOCIATION

6114 Highway 61
Little Marais, MN 55614
218-726-1443
www.purefood.com

RODALE INSTITUTE

611 Siegfriedale Road
Kutztown, PA 19530
800-823-6285
www.rodaleinstitute.org

USDA NATIONAL ORGANIC PROGRAM

www.ams.usda.gov/nop

ORGANIC ALLIANCE

400 Selby Ave, Suite T
St. Paul, MN 55102
651-265-3678
www.organic.org

environmental & campaign organizations

ENVIRONMENTAL DEFENSE

257 Park Avenue South
New York, NY 10010
800-684-3322
www.edf.org

CENTER FOR FOOD SAFETY

66 Pennsylvania Ave SE
Suite 302
Washington, DC 20003
202-547-9359
www.centerforfoodsafety.org

FOUNDATION ON ECONOMIC TRENDS

1660 L Street NW, Suite 216
Washington DC 20036
202-466-2823
www.biotechcentury.org

GREENPEACE USA

564 Mission Street
PO Box 416
San Francisco, CA 94105
800-326-0959
www.greenpeaceusa.org/ge/

FRIENDS OF THE EARTH (FOE)

1025 Vermont Ave NW
Washington, DC
20005-6303
phone: 202-783-7400;
877-843-8687
f: 202-783-0444
www.foe.org/safefood

CENTER FOR ETHICS AND TOXICS

39141 South Highway 1
P.O.Box 673
Gualala, CA 95445
704-884-1700
www.cetos.org

MOTHERS AND OTHERS FOR A LIVABLE PLANET

40 West 20th Street
New York, NY 10011-4211
212-242-0010
www.igc.apc.org/mothers

CAMPAIGN TO LABEL GENETICALLY ENGINEERED FOODS

PO Box 55699
Seattle, WA 98155
425-771-4049
www.thecampaign.org

UNION OF CONCERNED SCIENTISTS

2 Brattle Square
Cambridge, MA 02238-9105
617-547-5552
www.ucsusa.org

PEOPLE'S EARTH NETWORK

2192 Massachusetts Avenue
Cambridge, MA 02140
617-491-7646
www.peoplesearth.org

MOTHERS FOR NATURAL LAW

PO Box 1900
Fairfield, IA 52556
515-472-2040
www.safe-food.org

BIOENGINEERING ACTION NETWORK OF NORTH AMERICA

www.tao.ca/~ban/

CHEFS COLLABORATIVE

www.chefnet.com/cc2000

CITIZENS FOR HEALTH

800-357-2211
www.citizens.org

INSTITUTE OF SCIENCE IN SOCIETY (ISIS)

www.I-sis.dircon.co.uk

CONSUMERS UNION

101 Truman Ave
Yonkers, NY 10703
914-378-2452
www.consumersunion.org/food/food.htm

COUNCIL FOR RESPONSIBLE GENETICS

5 Upland Road, Suite 3
Cambridge, MA 02140
617-868-0870
www.gene-watch.org

RURAL ADVANCEMENT FOUNDATION INTERNATIONAL

PO Box 640
Pittsboro, NC 27319
www.fafi.org

THE EDMONDS INSTITUTE

20319 92nd Avenue West
Edmonds, WA 98020
425-775-5383
www.edmonds-institute.org

NATIONAL GEOGRAPHIC SOCIETY

1145 17th Street N.W.
Washington, DC 20036-4688

P.O. Box 98199
Washington, DC 20090-8199
www.nationalgeographic.com

THE SIERRA CLUB

85 Second St.
San Francisco, CA 94105-3441
www.sierraclub.org

certification bodies

INDEPENDENT ORGANIC INSPECTORS ASSOCIATION

PO Box 6
Broadus, MT 59317
406-436-2031
f:406-436-2031
www.ioia.net

CALFORNIA CERTIFIED ORGANIC FARMERS

1115 Mission Street
Santa Cruz, CA 95060
831-423-226
f: 831-423-4528
www.ccof.org

FARM VERIFIED ORGANIC

5449 45th Street SE
Medina, ND 58467
701-486-3578
f: 701-486-3580
www.tradecorridor.com/fvo
FVO is an interantional organic cerification organization.

NOFA/NEW YORK CERTIFICATON PROGRAM

26 Towpath Road
Binghamton, NY 13904
607-724-9851
f: 607-724-9853
NOFA/NY has a certification program that sets production standards and offers certification services in such varied areas as vegetables, livestock, wine, yogurt, greenhouse crops, and more.

NOVA SCOTIA ORGANIC GROWERS ASSOCIATON

PO Box 16
Annapolis Royal, NS
BOS 1NO
Canada
902-825-2432
f: 902-825-3139
www.gks.com/NSOGA

MIDWEST ORGANIC SERVICES ASSOCIATION, INC.

PO Box 344
Viroqua, WI 54665
608-734-3349
f: 608-734-3306
E-mail: mosa@mwt.net
MOSA provides organic cetification services for farmers, processors, on-farm processors, and grower groups in the Midwest.

ORGANIC CROP IMPROVEMENT ASSOCIATION

1001 Y Street, Suite B
Lincoln, NE 68508
402-477-2323
f: 402-477-4325
www.ocia.org
OCIA offers certification services for organic growers and processors around the world.

NORTH OKANAGAN ORGANIC ASSOCIATION

4607A 23rd Street
Vernon, BC V1T 4K7
Canada
250-260-4429
f: 250-260-4436
www.certifiedorganic.bc.ca

food & drink

AMERICAN CULINARY FEDERATION

301 E Street NW
Washington, DC 20049
904-824-4468
800-624-9458
f: 904-825-4758
www.acfchefs.org
ACF offers a host of educational programs including cooking, sanitation, supervisory development, and nutrition for chefs, cooks, and culinary professionalsb.

FOOD AND DRUG ADMINISTRATION (FDA)

5600 Fishers Lane
Rockville, MD 20857
301-443-3170
The FDA enforecs the Federal Food, Drug, and Cosmetics Act and related laws to ensure product purity.

U.S. FOOD CO-OP DIRECTORY

www.purefood.org/coopindex.ht

U.S. DEPARTMENT OF AGRICULTURE (USDA)

Independence Avenue and 14th Street NW
Washington, DC 20250
202-720-4323
Meat, poultry, fruits, and vegetables are inspected and approved by the USDA.

FARMER'S MARKETS

www.farmersmarketonline.com/index.html

USDA'S FARMER'S MARKET SOURCE

www.ams.usda.gov/farmersmarkets/

COMMUNITY SUPPORT

(resource page)
www.farmersmarketonline.com/Communit.htm

COOPERATIVE DEVELOPMENT INSTITUTE

277 Federal Street
Greenfield, MA 01301
413-774-7599

babycare

LA LECHE LEAGUE INTERNATIONAL

PO Box 1209
Franklin Park, IL 60131
800-LA-LECHE
www.lalecheleague.org

health & beauty

FOUNDATION FOR TOXIC-FREE DENTISTRY

PO Box 608010
Orlando, FL 32860-8010
Investigates and provides information on the biocompatibility of materials used in dentistry, particularly the health effects of mercury amalgam fillings.

gardening

AMERICAN COMMUNITY GARDEN NETWORK

100 N 20th St., 5th floor
Philadelphia, PA 19103-1495
215-988-8785
www.communitygarden.org/index.html

ACRES, USA

PO Box 8800
Metairie, LA 70011
504-889-2100

BIO-DYNAMIC FARMING AND GARDENING ASOCIATION

PO Box 550
Kimberton, PA 19442
610-935-7797

EPA PESTICIDE HOTLINE

800-858-7378

NORTHWEST COALITION FOR ALTERNATIVES TO PESTICIDES

PO Box 1393
Eugene, OR 97440
541-344-5044
Information on less toxic alternatives to pesticide hazards. Publishes the Journal of Pesticide Reform.

BIO-INTEGRAL RESOURCE CENTER

PO Box 7414
Berkeley, CA 94707
510-524-2567

recycling

OFFICE OF THE FEDERAL ENVIRONMENTAL EXECUTIVE

202-564-1297
mcpoland.fran@ofee.gov
Designed to expand and strengthen the Federal government's commitment to recycling and buying recycled content and environmentally preferable products, including biobased products.

GREENPEACE USA

1436 U Street, N.W.
Washington DC 20009
202-462-1177
USA@green2.greenpeace.org

THE ENVIRONMENT PROJECT

800 South Rolling Road
Catonsville MD 21228-5317
410-719-6551
cfox@neors,cat.cc.md.us
Provides wide range of credit, professional-development, grant-funded and outreach programs.

INSTITUTE FOR LOCAL SELF-RELIANCE

2425 18th St., N.W.
Washington DC 20009
202-232-4108
F: 202-332-0463
bplatt@ilsr.org
This is a nonprofit research and educational organization offering technical assistance on recycling and other sustainable development issues.

GREEN SEAL

1730 Rhode Island Ave,
NW, Suite 1050
Washington DC 20036-3101
202-331-7337
F: 1-202-331-7533
Environmental labeling organization that awards a "Green Seal of Approval" to products that cause less environmental harm than similar products.

AIR & WASTE MANAGEMENT ASSOCIATION

One Gateway Center,
Third Floor
Pittsburgh PA 15222
412-232-3444
F: 412-232-3450
swalsh@awma.org
The Air & Waste Management Association promotes global environmental responsibility.

EARTH DAY NETWORK

91 Marion St.
Seattle WA 98104
206-264-0114 ext. 226
mackermann@earthday.net
Promotes Earth Day events around the world.

EARTH SHARE

3400 International Drive,
NW Suite 2K
Washington DC 20008
800-875-3863
robin@earthshare.org
Federation of top environmental and conservation agencies, working together to protect global environmenal, health, and natural resources through workplace giving and public education.

GRASSROOTS RECYCLING NETWORK

PO Box 49283
Athens GA 30604-9283
706-613-7121
zerowaste@grrn.org
Works for corporate responsibility for waste, government policies for resource conservation, and sustainable jobs from discards.

WORLD WATCH INSTITUTE

1776 Massachusetts Ave., NW
Washington, DC 20036-1904
202-452-1999
worldwatch@worldwatch.org
Dedicated to fostering the evolution of an environmentally sustainable society through the conduct of inter-disciplinary nonpartisan research on emerging global environmental issues, the results of which are widely disseminated throughout the world.

ENVIRONMENTAL RECYCLING, INC.

P.O.Box 92229
Anchorage, AK 99509-2229
907-243-8577
glass@pobox.alaska.net
Concerned with many aspects of processing and recycling glass and related materials.

GLOBAL RECYCLING NETWORK

www.grn.com
GRN provides a local, national, and international directory of recycling organizations.

ENVIRONMENTAL DEFENSE FUND

257 Park Avenue South
New York, NY 10010
800-684-3322
*From water to wildlife, from
toxic chemicals to tropical
rainforests, EDF chooses the
important areas where people
can make a difference in
defending the environment.*

ENVIRONMENTAL RECYCLING, INC.

P.O.Box 92229
Anchorage, AK 99509-2229
907-243-8577
glass@pobox.alaska.net
*Concerned with many
aspects of processing and
recycling glass and related
materials.*

petcare

AMERICAN HOLISTIC VETERINARY MEDICAL ASSOCIATION

2214 Old Emmorton Road
Bel Air, MD 21015
410-569-0795

*A professional organization
of veterinarians who use
nontraditional techniques,
including alternative
nutrition, homeopathy, and
acupuncture.*

What to read

general

directories

National Organic Directory Community Alliance with Family Farmers (CAFF)
PO Box 363
Davis CA 95617-9900
530-756-8518
f: 530-756-7857
www.caff.org
Published annually. This directory reaches an international audience and provides information on farmers, wholesalers, manufacturers/processors, and retailers. It also provides information on support businesses, certifcation groups, resource groups, and farm suppliers. Listings provide company and organization names, addresses, contact numbers, and contact people. Resources are listed regionally as well as nationally.

The Organic Pages
Organic Trade Association
OTA Press
Organic Trade Association's 1998 North American Resource Directory; 272 pages, spiral bound. This volume provides comprehensive contact information for over 770 OTA members as well as listings for over 530 certified organic farms in North America. THE ORGANIC PAGES contains detailed organic industry information on an enormous range of businesses.

Natural Resource Directory: The Healthy Yellow Pages
520 Washington Blvd
Suite 509
Marina del Rey, CA 90292
www.nrd.com
The Healthy Yellow Pages is published biannualy and serves health-conscious consumers in Los Angeles, Orange, Riverside, San Bernardino, and Ventura counties.

books

Carson, Rachel
Silent Spring
(Houghton Mifflin, 1962, repr. Penguin, 1999)

Cummins, Ronnie Lilliston, Ben
Genetically Engineered Food: A Self-Defense Guide For Consumers
(Marlowe & Company, 2000)

Fincher, Cynthia
Healthy Living in a Toxic World
(Colorado Springs, CO: Pinon Press, 1996)

Gosslin, R.E. et al.
The Clinical Toxicology of Consumer Products
(Baltimore: The Williams & Wilkins Company, 1984)

magazines & newsletters

The Green Guide
Mothers & Others for a Livable Planet
40 W. 20th Street 9th Floor
New York, NY 10011
212-242-0010

NewAge Journal
PO Box 52375
Boulder, CO 80321-3275
800-234-4556

Natural Health
PO Box 57329
Boulder, CO 80322-7320
800-666-8576
This bimonthly "guide to well-being" contains information on natural healing, with natural living.

Safe Home Resource Guide
PO Box 3420
Westport, CT 06880
203-227-1276

Spectrum
Spectrum Universal Corp.
2702-D Camellia Street
Durham, NC 27705
919-383-6492

Sierra
The Sierra Club Magazine
Sierra
P.O. Box 52968
Boulder, CO 80328.
www.sierraclub.org
Published bimonthly, Sierra is the official magazine of the Sierra Club. Annual dues are $35. Members of the Sierra Club subscribe to Sierra through $7.50 of their dues.

National Geographic Magazine
Magazine Orders
P.O. Box 63002
Tampa, Florida 33663-3002
www.nationalgeographic.com

Yoga Journal
2054 University Avenue
Suite 600
Berkeley, CA 94704
415-841-9200

food & drink

books

Blythman, Joanna
The Food We Eat
(Penguin, 1998)

Elliott, Renee & Treuille, Eric
Organic Cookbook
(Dorling Kindersley, 2000)

Mothers & Others For a Livable Planet
The Green Kitchen Handbook
40 West 20th Street,
9th floor
New York, NY 10011
212-242-0545

Mott, Lawrie & Snyder, Karen of the Natural Defense Council
Pesticide Alert: A Guide to Pesticides in Fruits and Vegetables
(San Francisco: Sierra Club Books, 1987)

Johnson, Robert
The Consumer's Guide to Organic Wine
(Pasichnyk, 1993)

Marlin, John Tepper, Ph.D.
The Catalog of Healthy Food
(New York: Bantam Books, 1990)

Rohe, Fred
Nature's Kitchen: The Complete Guide to the New American Diet
(Storey Communications, 1986)

Rodale & Staff
Prevention's Healthy Cook
(Rodale Press, 2000)

Wargo, John
Our Children's Toxic Legacy
(Yale University Press, 1996)

Watterson, Andrew
Pesticides and Your Food: How to Reduce the Risks to Your Health
(London: Green Print, 1991)

Weir, David & Shapiro, Mark
Circle of Poison: Pesticides and People in a Hungry World
(Institute for Food and Development Policy, 1981)

Winter, Ruth
A Consumer Dictionary of Food Additives
(Crown Publishers, 1989)

magazines

Natural Life Magazine
RR 1,
St. George
Ontario, Canada N0E 1N0
800-215-9574
natural@life.ca
www.life.ca/index.html

www.ecowine.com
A monthly e-zine by the San Francisco-based Organic Wine Company is always entertaining and informative, and some of the wines it lists can be found in the UK, too.

baby care

Chae, Jayni
Blueprint for a Greeen School
(Scholastic, 1995)

Green, Nancy Sokol
Poisoning Our Children: Surviving in a Toxic World
(The Noble Press, 1991)

Kenda, Margaret Elizabeth & Williams, Phyllis S.
The Natural Baby Food Cookbook
(Avon Books 1982)

Lanski, Vicki
Baking Soda: Over 500 Fabulous, Fun, and Frugal Uses You've Probably Never Thought of
(The Book Peddlers, 1995)

Mothering magazine
PO Box 1690
Santa Fe, NM 87504
505-984-8116

Rapp, Doris, M.D.
Is This Your Child? Discovering and Treating Unrecognized Allergies
(William Morrow, 1991)

Schoemaker, Joyce M. Ph.D.
Healthy Homes, Healthy Kids: Protecting Your Children From Everyday Environmental Hazards
(Island Press, 1991)

Weed, Susan S.
WiseWoman Herbal for the Childbearing Years
(Ash Tree Publishing, 1986)

Vann, Lizzie
Organic Baby & Toddler Cookbook (Dorling Kindersley, 2000)

health & beauty

Miller, Susan
The Natural Soap Book: Making Herbal and Vegetable-based Soaps
(Storey Communications, 1995)

Steinman, David & Epstein, Samuel S., MD
The Safe Shopper's Bible
(Simon & Schuster, 1994)

Tourles, Stephanie
The Herbal Body Book: A Natural Approach to Healthier Hair, Skin, and Nails
(Storey Communications, 1994)

Weschler, Toni
Taking Charge of Your Fertility: The Definitive Guide To Natural Birth Control and Pregnancy Achievement
(HarperPerennial, 1996)

Winter, Ruth
A Consumer's Directory of Cosmetic Ingredients
(Three Rivers Press, 1999)

gardening
books

Appelhof, Mary
Worms Eat My Garbage
(Flower Press, 1982)

Bartholomew, Mel
Square Foot Gardening
(Rodale Press, 1981)

Franklin, Stuart
Building a Healthy Lawn
(Storey Communications, 1988)

Coleman, Eliot
The New Organic Grower: A Master's Manual of Tools and Techniques for the Home and Market Gardner
(Chelsea Green, 1996)

Grainger, Janette & Moore, Connie
Natural Insect Repellents: for Pets, People & Plants
(The Herb Bar, 1991)

Greenwood, Pippa
Pippa's Organic Kitchen Garden (Dorling Kindersley, 1999)

Hamilton, Geoff
The Organic Garden Book
(Dorling Kindersley, 1987)

Kourik, Robert
Designing and Maintaining Your Edible Lanscape Naturally
(Metamorphic Press, 1986)

Olkowski, William
Common Sense Pest Control: Least-toxic Solutions for Your Home, Garden, Pets, and Community
(Taunton Press, 1991)

Pest Publications
Shepherd's Purse: Organic Pest Control Handbook
(The Book Publishing Company, 1987)

Schultz, Warren
The Chemical-Free Lawn
(Rodale Press, 1989)

Philbrick, Helen & Gregg, Richard
Companion Plants and How to Use Them
(Devin-Adair, 1966)

Pleasant, Barbara
The Gardener's Bug Book: Earth-safe Insect Control
(Storey Communications, 1994)

Schultz, Warren
The Chemical-Free Lawn
(Rodale Press, 1989)

Starcher, Allison Mia
Good Bugs for Your Garden
(Algonquin Books, 1995)

Stein, Dan
Dan's Practical Guide to Least Toxic Home Pest Control
(Hulogosi Communication, 1991)

magazines

Biological Urban Gardening Services (BUGS)
PO Box 76
Citrus Heights, CA 95611-0076
916-726-5377

Common Sense Pest Control Quarterly
Bio-Integral Resource Center
PO Box 7414
Berkeley, CA 94707
510-524-2567
www.birc.org

Fine Gardening
The Taunton Press
PO Box 5506
Newtown, CT 06470-5506
800-283-7252

Kitchen Garden
The Taunton Press
PO Box 5506
Newtown, CT 06470-5506
800-283-7252

Organic Gardening
Rodale Press
33 East Minor Street,
Emmaus, PA
800-666-2206
www.organicgardening.com

home & office
directories and newsletters

Interior Concerns
PO Box 2386
Mill Valley, CA 94942
415-389-8049
A bimonthly newsletter that provids information for designers, architects, builders, and homeowners on environmental products, issues, and industry changes.

Global Recycling Network
www.grn.com

Buy Smart, Buy Safe: A Consumer Guide to Less-Toxic Products
Washington Toxics Coalition
4516 University Way NE
Seattle, WA 98105
206-632-1545
wtc@igc.apc.org

Interior Concerns Resource Guide
PO Box 2386
Mill Valley, CA 94942
415-389-8049
This resource guide lists products, manufacturers, consultants, and other resources.

books

Berthold-Bond, Annie
Clean & Green: The Complete Guide to Nontoxic and Environmentally Safe Household Cleaning
(Ceres Press, 1990)

Jacobsen, Lauren
Children's Art Hazards
(Natural Resources Defense Council)

McCann, Michael
Artist Beware: The Hazards and Precautions in Working with Art and Craft Materials
(Watson Guptill Publications, 1979)

Pearson, David
The Natural House Catalog: Everything You Need to Create an Environmentally Friendly Home
(Simon & Schuster, 1996)

petcare

Anderson, Nina, & Peiper, Howard
Are You Poisoning Your Pets? A Guidebook on How Our Lifestyles Affect the Health of Our Pets
(Safe Goods, 1996)

De Bairacli Levy, Juliette
The Complete Herbal Handbook for the Dog and Cat
(Faber & Faber, 1991)

Frazier, Anitra
The New Natural Cat: A Complete Guide for Finicky Owners
(Penguin Books, 1990)

Goldstein, Martin
The Nature of Animal Healing: the Path to Our Pet's Health, Happiness, and Longevity
(Alfred A. Knopf, 1999)

Lazarus, Pat
Keep Your Pet Healthy the Natural Way
(Keats Publishing, 1999)

Patmore, Angela
Your Natural Dog: A Guide to Behavior and Health Care
(Carroll & Graf, 1993)

Pitcairn, Richard H., & Hubble Pitcairn, Susan
Dr. Pitcairn's Complete Guide to Natural Health for Dogs and Cats
(Rodale Press, 1995)

Puotinen, C.J.
The Encyclopedia of Natural Pet Care
(Keats Publishing Inc. 1998)

finance

Environmental Capital Network
416 Longshore Drive
Ann Arbor MI 48105
313-996-8387
F: 313-996-8732
E-mail: ecn@BizServe.com
ECN introduces environmental and green technology companies raising capital to angels, venture-capital firms, and private equity investors.

Where to buy

general organic retailers

To shop at an organic retailer, be it an organic supermarket or farm shop, or one specializing in organic and green products for your home or baby, is to enter a different world giving a special experience that will keep you coming back time and time again. In them you can shop sustainably and spend your money in positive ways, choosing products that have an ethical clean bill of health and are good for you and good for the planet.

Organic supermarket chains and independent organic shops stock everything you need for organic living – food, drink, petfoods, natural and organic healthcare, and eco-friendly household goods and other products. None stock any genetically modified products. The atmosphere is fun and personalized, and there are friendly and knowledgeable staff eager to give you whatever organic advice you need.

You can also shop for all your organic needs through mail order or online. There are home delivery services that deliver a range of organic food and "green" nonfood products. If you want to know where your nearest organic retailers are located, consult one of the organic directories. Alternatively, organic websites provide lists of local organic growers and stores in your area.

supermarkets & general stores

MOTHER'S MARKET & KITCHEN

225 East 17th Street
Costa Mesa, CA 92627
(locations in Costa Mesa, Irvine, Huntington Beach and Laguna Hills)
949-548-7786
Since 1978, this natural food market, restaurant, deli, and juice bar has provided outstanding quality and selection in organic produe and foods.

HUNGRY HOLLOW CO-OP

841 Chestnut Ridge Road
Chestnut Ridge, NY 10977
914-356-3319
f: 914-356-3954
Hungry Hollow Co-op carries a full line of organic produce, dairy, bakery, and packaged products and homemade foods.

LIFETHYME COMPLETE NATURAL MARKET

410 Sixth Avenue
Greenwich Village, NY
212-420-9009
2275 Broadway
New York, NY
212-721-9000

LA MONTANITA CO-OP NATURAL FOODS MARKET

3500 Central SE
Nob Hill Shopping Center
Albuquerque, NM 87106
505-265-4631
www.lamontanita.com
La Monanita Co-op is a member-owned natural foods grocery store that offers natural and organic foods, supplements, and body care.

mail order & online

DEER VALLEYFARM

RD 1, Box 173
Guilford, NY 13780
607-764-8556

DIAMOND ORGANICS

Freedom,CA 95089
800-922-2396

GOLD MINE NATURAL FOOD COMPANY

3419 Hancock Street
San Diego, CA 92110-4307
800-475-FOOD

JAFFE BROTHERS

PO Box 636
Valley Center, CA
92082-0636
619-749-1133

MOTHER'S MARKET & KITCHEN

225 East 17th Street
Costa Mesa, CA 92627
949-548-7786

mail order & online

The organic sector is better served than most, with several well-established mail order and online companies providing food and drink, and others providing eco-necessities, including household products, bodycare, babycare, natural remedies, and clothes. Some offer a wide range of organic and eco-friendly products from food to hardware. You can expect a high level of professionalism and friendly, efficient service.

Mail order and online shopping are modern, convenient ways to shop. They cut down on car journeys, are less stressful, and leave you more quality time. They mean saying goodbye to battling in lines and carrying heavy bags, and let you shop in a leisurely way, when you are relaxed.

THE KNOW-HOW

❖ Phone around or browse the internet and get details of several companies to see which ones are likely to suit you best. Prices and services can vary, so compare these and see what you are getting for your money.

❖ Check out the small print, what happens if orders go astray, and ordering days and deadlines.

❖ Do not be afraid to get advice and ask as many questions as you want to.

❖ If ordering regularly, get to know one person who can deal with your order every time you use the service.

❖ New websites are constantly being developed and updated. To ensure accessibility, make sure you are using the latest browser software. Many online companies include these on their websites for you to download free of charge.

❖ Companies' websites and e-mail addresses are listed throughout the directory.

food & drink

Shopping for organic food and drink is easy – choose from the various options listed here and mix and match to suit. For example, you can shop in a supermarket for your basics, subscribe to a local box program for fresh produce, and have the convenience of mail order for meat. You can do all your organic shopping online if you prefer, go local and visit a farmers' market, or plan a trip to an organic supermarket or store to discover for yourself what a pleasure shopping organically can be.

major retailers

All major supermarkets stock organic essentials, including drinks, baby foods, chilled and frozen foods, and, increasingly, ready-made meals, although the selection varies from store to store and some chains sell far less than others.

health & wholefood shops

These stock a wide line of pantry basics such as dried foods, biscuits, canned soups and beans, breakfast cereals, soy products, juices, jams, oils, and often dairy products. Some sell fresh produce. They usually stock eco-friendly household products.

go local

Buying organic food from local producers enables you to enjoy the freshest produce, gives the best value and the most satisfaction, helps to support local economies, and cuts down on food miles. There are many local initiatives in towns and cities (*see page 38*), including farmers' markets (*see below*).

farmers' markets

These benefit farmers, consumers, the community, and the environment. Hundreds are held, daily or on weekends, all over the country. The markets are not necessarily organic but sell locally-produced foods, including those from organic producers. Some also have family entertainment and craft stalls.

THE KNOW-HOW

❖ Markets operate within fixed hours, and they often open for business very early in the morning. Inclement weather may be a factor in enabling some of the vendors to set up at a market. It is best to check dates, details, and opening times before you go.
❖ Check out public transportation, proximity to a parking lot, and whether the market is covered or at least partially so.

❖ For the best selection, go as early as you can.
❖ Take enough cash and small change and a large shopping bag. In summer, an insulated box can be useful.
❖ Have a good look around before you buy. Talk to people, ask as many questions as you want, and accept tastings.

WHAT CAN YOU BUY?

At farmers' markets, no produce may be bought in, and produce may be required to be grown, bred, caught, pickled, brewed, or baked by the merchants themselves. Often the varieties of fruit and vegetables for sale will be locally produced, the meat will come from rare breeds, and there will be seasonal delights such as turnip tops, or local treats that are a rarity elsewhere.

farmers' markets

Farmers' markets are the ultimate local shopping experience and a return to how markets used to be: farmers selling their own produce direct to the consumer (*see page 38*).

farm shops

These range from very small shops selling farm produce to those that sell everything, have farm trails and a café, and provide a focus for the local community. Business hours vary, so call first to check.

COMMUNITY SUPPORT
www.farmersmarketonline.com/Community.htm

FARMER'S MARKETS
www.farmersmarketonline.com/index.html

MISSOURI ALTERNATIVES CENTER
agebb.missouri.edu/mac/

URBAN AGRICULTURE NOTES/CITY FARMER CANADA'S OFFICE OF URBAN AGRICULTURE
www.cityfarmer.org

NEW MEXICO FARMERS MARKETING ASSOCIATION
www.farmersmarketsnm.org

THE SMALL FARM PROGRAM USDA-COOPERATIVE STATE RESEARCH, EDUCATION AND EXTENSION SERVICE
www.reeusda.gov/smallfarm

SUSTAINABLE AGRICULTURE NETWORK
www.sare.org

USDA'S FARMER'S MARKET SOURCE
www.ams.usda.gov/farmersmarkets/

meat

ALASKA NATURAL BEEF
Bering Pacific Ranch
Umnak Island
Box 326
Unalaska, AK 99685
888-384-5366
www.alaskanatural.com

COLEMAN NATURAL PRODUCTS INC.
5140 Race Court
Denver, CO 80216
303-297-9393
www.colemanmeats.com

DEER VALLEYFARM
RD 1, Box 173
Guilford, NY 13780
607-764-8556

EBERLY POULTRY FARMS
1095 Mount Airy Road
Stevens, PA 17578
717-336-6905
www.eberlypoultry.com

LAURA'S LEAN BEEF
2285 Executive Drive
Suite 200
Lexington, KY 40505
606-299-7707
800-487-5326
www.laurasleanbeef.com

ORGANIC VALLEY FAMILY OF FARMS CROPP COOPERATIVE
507 W. Main Street
La Farge, WI 54639
888-444-6455
ww.organicvalley.com

WALNUT ACRES
Penns Creek, PA 17862
717-837-0601

WHIPPOORWILL FARM
Lakevill, CT 06039-0717
203-435-9657

WOLFE'S NECK FARM
10 Burnett Road
Freeport, ME 04032

fish

WALNUT ACRES
Penns Creek, PA 17862
717-837-0601

WOLFE'S NECK FARM
10 Burnett Road
Freeport, ME 04032

dairy

CZIMER FOODS
13136 W. 159th Street
Lockport, IL 60441
708-301-7152

DEER VALLEYFARM
RD 1, Box 173
Guilford, NY 13780
607-764-8556

DUTCH MILL CHEESE SHOP
2001 N. State Road 1
Cambridge City, IN 47327
317-478-5847

GOODNESS GREENESS
5959 South Lowe
Chicago, IL 60621
773-224-4411
www.goodnessgreeness.com

SHELBURNE FARMS
Shelburne, VT 05482
802-985-8686

VIROQUA FOOD COOPERATIVE
303 North Center Avenue
Viroqua, WI 54665
608-637-7511

WOLFE'S NECK FARM
10 Burnett Road
Freeport, ME 04032

flour, bread & baked goods

FIDDLER'S GREEN FARM
800 729 7935
www.fiddlersgreenfarm.com

RUDI'S BAKERY
3640 Walnut Street
Boulder, CO 80301
303-447-0495
www.rudisbakery.com

SUNORGANIC FARM
Box 2429
Valley Center, CA 92082
888-269-9888
www.sunorganic.com

herbs & spices

ALTERNATIVES FROM NATURE BY RAIN BEAR
148 S. Broad Street
Lititz, PA 17534
717-627-1077
www.herbsrainbear.com

FRONTIER NATURAL PRODUCTS CO-OP
800-786-1388
www.frontierherb.com

oils

CALIFORNIA OLIVE OIL
134 Canal Street
Salem, MA 01970
978-745-7840
www.olive-oil.com

SADEC ORGANIC
PO Box 1246
Modesto, CA 95353
800-551-9612
wwwsadeorganic.com

tea & coffee

KALANI ORGANIC
800-200-4377
www.kalanicoffee.com

SATORI ORGANIC HERBAL TEAS
800-729-7935
www.fiddlersgreenfarm.com

wines & juices

Many supermarkets now offer something in the way of organic wine, but some selections are better than others. For a wider choice – and knowledgable service – try these specialists, and let them deliver!

CF FRESH
922 3rd Street
P.O. Box 665
Sedro-Woolley, WA 98284
360-855-0566
www.rootbaga.com
a range of organic juices

GREAT FERMENTATIONS
87 Larkspur Street
San Rafael, CA 94901
800-570-2337

ORGANIC WINE COMPANY
1592 Union Street, #350
San Francisco, CA 94123
888-ECO-WINE (326-9463)
www.ecowine.com

babycare

AFTER THE STORK
PO Box 44321
Rio Rancho, NM
87174-4321
800-441-4775
505-867-7000
*Babies' and kids' clothing
and sun protection*

ALLERGY RESOURCES
PO Box 444
Guffey, CO 80820
800-USE-FLAX
*Diapers, bedding, laundry
products, and more*

BABY BUNZ & COMPANY
PO Box 113
Lynden, WA 98264
800-676-4559

BIOBOTTOMS
PO Box 6069
Petaluma, CA 94953
707-778-7945
*Babies' and kids' clothing
and diapers*

BRIGHT FUTURE FUTON
3120 Central Avenue SE
Albuquerque, NM 87106
505-268-9738
Bedding and cribs

DECENT EXPOSURES
PO Box 27206
Seattle, WA 98125
800-505-4949
Baby food and clothing

**EARTH'S BEST BABY
FOOD**
Middlebury, VT

FOR KEEPS FRIENDS
217 SW "C" Avenue #190
Lawton, OK 73501
Toys

GARNET HILL
Box 262 Main Street
Franconia, NH 03580-0262
800622-6216

HEARTHSONG
6519 N. Galena Road
Peoria, IL 61656-1773
800325-2502

LOGONA USA
12 Wall Street
Asheville, NC 28801
800-252-9630
Baby-care products

MOTHERWEAR
320 Riverside Drive
Northampton, MA 01060
800-950-2500

ORGANIC COTTONS
103 Hoffecker Road
Phoenixville, PA 19460
610-495-9986

**OSTHEIMER WOODEN
TOYS**
PO Box 407
Wyoming, RI 02898
800-249-9090

WELEDA
PO Box 769
Spring Valley, NY 10977
914-352-6145
Baby-care products

gardening

ACRES U.S.A.
PO Box 9547
Kansas City, MO 64113
816-737-0064
pesticides

AGACCESS
PO Box 2008
Davis, CA 95617
916-756-7177
pesticides

**BIO-ORGANICS HOME
GARDENER CENTER**
3200 Corte Malpaso #107
Camarillo, CA 93102
800-604-0444
**www.chappyspowerorganic
s.com**

BOUNTIFUL GARDENS
18001 Shafer Ranch Road
Willits, CA 95490-9626
707-459-6410
www.bountifulgardens.com
*Specializing in seed with a
focus on biointensive
farming and gardening. Also
small quantities of hard-to-
find covercrop seed.*

GARDENER'S SUPPLY
128 Intervale Raod
Burlington, VT 15401-2804
800-863-1700
*pesticides, insect repellents,
lawn care*

GARDENS ALIVE!
5100 Schenley Place
Lawrenceburg, IN 47025
812-537-8650
www.gardens-alive.com
*flea control, garden
pesticides, lawn care*

GREEN BAN
PO Box 146
Norway, IA 52318
insect repellents

**HARMONY FARM
SUPPLY**
PO Box 460
Graton, CA 95444
707-823-9125
www.harmonyfarm.com
pesticides

HORIZON HERBS
PO Box 69
Williams, OR 97544
541-846-6704
**www.chatlink.com/~herbse
ed/**

**THE INVISIBLE
GARDENER**
PO Box 4311
Malibu, CA 90265
310-457-4438
www.invisiblegardener.com
*natural pest control
and more.*

**LEDDEN BROTHERS,
INC.**
195 Center Avenue
PO Box 7
Sewell, NJ 08080-0007
888-783-733
www.leddens.com

**THE NATIONAL
GARDENING COMPANY**
217 San Anselmo Avenue
San Anselmo, CA 94960
415-456-5060
pesticides

NITRON INDUSTRIES
PO Box 1447
Fayetteville, AR 72702
800-835-0123
www.nitron.com
*organic fertilizers, soil
amendments, nonhybrid
seeds, and more.*

**ORGANIC GROWERS
SUPPLY**
PO Box 520
Waterville, ME 04903
207-873-7333

**PEACEFUL VALLEY
FARM SUPPLY**
PO Box 2209
Grass Valley, CA 95945
916-272-4769
www.groworganic.com
pesticides

PLANET NATURAL
1612 Gold Avenue
PO Box 3146
Bozeman, MT 59772
406-587-5891
800-289-6656
www.planetnatural.com
natural pest controls

health & beauty

Not every ingredient in these companies' products may be natural, but these are the companies that are making real efforts to use fewer synthetic ingredients and more organically produced ingredients, rather than using "natural" and "organic" merely as a marketing ploy.

ALLERGY RELIEF SHOP
3371 Whittle Springs Raod
Knoxville, TN 37917
800-626-2810

AMERICAN ENVIRONMENTAL HEALTH FOUNDATION
9345 Walnut Hill Lane
Suite 225
Dallas, TX
800-428-2343

ALEXANDRA AVERY
4717 SE Belmont Street
Portland, OR 97215
800-669-1863

GOLD MINE NATURAL FOOD COMPANY
3419 Hancock Street
San Diego, CA 92110-4307
800-475-FOOD

JANICE CORPORATION
198 Route 46
Budd Lake, NJ 07828
800-526-4237

KAREN'S NONTOXIC PRODUCTS
1839 Dr. Jack Road
Conowingo, MD 21918
410-378-4936

KETTLE CARE
710 Trap Road
Columbia Falls, MT 59912
406-892-3294

THE LIVING SOURCE
PO Box 20155
Waco, TX 76702
800-662-8787

LOGONA USA
12 Wall Street
Asheville, NC 28801
800-648-6654

NATURAL LIFESTYLE
16 Lookout Drive
Asheville, NC 28804-3330
800-752-2775

SIMMONS HANDCRAFTS
42295 N. Highway 36
Bridgeville, CA 95526
707-777-1920

SUN PRECAUTIONS
2815 Wetmore Avenue
Everett, WA 98201
800-882-7860

TRADITIONAL PRODUCTS COMPANY
PO Box 564
Creswell, OR 97426
503-895-2957

WELEDA
PO Box 769
Spring Valley, NY 10977
914-352-6145

WOMANKIND
PO Box 1775
Sebastopol, CA 95473
707-522-8662

home & office

building supplies

U.S. GREEN BUILDING COUNCIL
1825 I Street NW
Suite 400
Washington, DC 20006
202-429-2081

The USGBC is a nonprofit consensus coalition of the building industry that promotes the understanding, development, and accelerated implementation of "green building" policies, programs technologies, standards, and design practices on a national basis.

furniture

GRATEFUL THREADS
1301 Spruce Street
Boulder, CO 80302
Beds and bedding

BRIGHT FUTURE FUTON
3120 Central Avenue SE
Alburquerque, NM 87106
505-268-9738
Beds, cribs, furniture

HEART OF VERMONT
PO Box 612
Barre, VT 05641
800-639-4123
Beds, bedding, cribs.

THE NATURAL BEDROOM
175 N. Main Street
Sebastopol, CA 95472
800-365-6563
Beds, bedding, and cribs

ROYAL-PEDIC
119 N. Fairfax Avenue
Los Angeles,
CA 90036
213-932-6155
Beds and bedding

SAJAMA ALPACA
PO Box 209
Ashland, OR 97520
541-488-3949
*Beds and bedding, carpeting,
flooring, yarns, fabrics,
and notions.*

SHAKER WORKSHOPS
PO Box 8001
Ashburnham, MA 01430-
8001
508-827-9900
Furniture

**SHAKER WORKSHOPS
WEST**
PO Box 487
Inverness, CA 94937
415-669-7256
Furniture

SOFA U LOVE
11948 San Vicente
Brentwood, CA 90049
310-207-2540
Furniture

**WILLSBORO WOOD
PRODUCTS**
PO Box 509
Keeseville, NY 12944
800-342-3373
Furniture

paints
& finishes

AFM ENTERPRISES
350 W. Ash Street
Suite 700
San Diego, CA 92101
619-239-0321

EARTH STUDIO
6761 Sebastopol Avenue
Suite 8
Sebastopol, CA 95472
707-823-2569

**ENVIRONMENTAL HOME
CENTER**
1724 4th Avenue
Seattle, WA 98134
800-281-9785

**OLD-FASHIONED MILK
PAINT COMPANY**
PO Box 222
Groton, MA 01450
508-448-6336

SINAN COMPANY
PO Box 857
Davis, CA 95617-0857
916-753-3104

reclaimed
materials

**ASSOCIATION FOR
RESOURCE
CONSERVATION, INC.**
P.O. Box 231
Centerport, NY 11721
631-757-0894
Fax: 1-631-757-0896
arclink@juno.com

*Maintains a materials
exchange site — Link-Ups
— to network available and
usable commercial by-
products, scrap, and reusable
items from businesses on
Long Island, New York, to
potential users.*

**FLORIDA ORGANICS
RECYCLERS
ASSOCIATION**
1015 US Highway 301 South
Tampa, FL 33619
813-681-0087
FORAinc@aol.com
*The Florida Organics
Recyclers Association is a
broad-based nonprofit
organization that offers an
opportunity to become
involved in all aspects of
organic materials recovery in
Florida.*

**VERMONT RETROWORKS
(ACCAG)**
282 Boardman Street
Middlebury VT 05753
877-292-9326
Fax: 877-292-9326
retroworks@mail.com

flooring

AFM ENTERPRISES
350 W. Ash Street
Suite 700
San Diego, CA 92101
619-239-0321

ALLEGRO RUG WEAVING
802 S. Sherman Drive
Longmont, CO 80501
800-783-1784

**ANDERSON
LABORATORIES**
PO Box 323
Witartford, VT 05084
802-295-7344

CAROUSEL CARPETS
1 Carousel Lane
Ukiah, CA 95482
704-485-0333

**COLIN CAMPBELL &
SONS**
1428 West Seventh Avenue
Vancouver BC
Canada V6H1C1
604-734-2758
800-677-5001 (USA)

DELLINGER
1943 N. Broad
Rome, GA 30161
706-291-7402

**HENDRICKSEN'S
NATURLICH**
PO Box 1677
Sebastopol, CA 95473
707-824-0914

THE NATURAL CHOICE
1365 Rufina Circle
Santa Fe, NM 87505
800-621-2591

SAJAMA ALPACA
PO Box 1209
Ashland, OR 97520
541-488-3949

cleaning products

ALLERGY RESOURCES
PO Box 444
Guffey, CO 80820
800-USE-FLAX

AMERICAN ENVIRONMENTAL HEALTH FOUNDATION
8345 Walnut Hill Lane
Suite 225
Dallas, TX 75231-4262
800-428-2343
214-361-9515

CAL BEN SOAP COMPANY
9828 Pearmain Street
Oakland, CA 94108
510-638-7092

GRANNY'S OLD-FASHIONED PRODUCTS
PO Box 660037
Arcadia, CA 91006
800-366-1762

JANICE CORPORATION
198 Route 46
Budd Lake, NJ 07828
800-526-4237

KAREN'S NONTOXIC PRODUCTS
1839 Dr. Jack Road
Conowingo, MD 21918
410-378-4936

THE LIVING SOURCE
PO Box 20155
Waco, TX 76702
800-662-8787

LOGONA USA
12 Wall Street
Asheville, NC 28801
800-648-6654

THE NATURAL CHOICE
1365 Rufina Circle
Santa Fe, NM 87505
800-621-2591

NONTOXIC ENVIRONMENTS
PO Box 384
Newmarket, NJ 03857
800-789-4348

REAL GOODS
555 Leslie Street
Ukiah, CA 95482-5507
800-762-7325

SEVENTH GENERATION
49 Hercules Drive
Colchester, VT 05446-1672
800-456-1177

SOAPWORKS
14450 Griffin Street
San Leandro, CA 94577
800-699-9917

water conservation

WATERWISER
6666 West Quincy Avenue
Denver, CO 80235
800-559-9855
www.waterwiser.org
WaterWiser is a program of the American Water Works Association operated in cooperation with the U.S. Bureau of Reclamation. The website contains a directory for water management service and product companies across the U.S. and Canada.

clothing & fabric

AMERICAN ENVIRONMENTAL HEALTH FOUNDATION
8345 Walnut Hill Lane
Suite 225
Dallas, TX 75231-4262
800-428-2343
214-361-9515

BARBARA COOLE DESIGNS
2631 Piner Road
Santa Rosa, CA 95401
800-992-8924
73003.1246@Compuserve.com

CASCO BAY FINE WOOLENS
34 Danforth Street
Portland, ME 04101
800-788-9842

CASTLE GRAY
PO Box 647
Manitou Springs, CO 80829
800-987-3747

CHIPANTS
120 Rising Road
Mill Valley, CA 94941
415-381-2407
www.chipants.com

THE CORDWAINER SHOP
67 Candia Road
Deerfield, NH 03037
603-463-7742
Footwear and shoe care

COTTON CLOUDS MAIL-ORDER YARNS
5176 S. 14Th Avenue
Dept NT
Safford, AZ 85546
800-322-7888
Fabrics, yarns, and notions

COTTON THREADS CLOTHING
Route 2, Box 90
Halletsville, TX 77964
409-562-2153
micyn@cvtv.net

THE COTTON PLACE
PO Box 7715
Waco, TX 76714
800-451-8866

EDDIE BAUER
PO Box 3700
Seattle, WA 98124-3700
800-426-8020

GARNET HILL
Box 262 Main Street
Franconia, NH 03580-0262
800-622-6216

GREEN MOUNTAIN SPINNERY
PO Box 54
Putney, VT 05346
802-587-4528

HEART OF VERMONT
PO Box 612
Barre, VT 05641
800-639-4123

HENDRICKSEN'S NATURLICH
PO Box 1677
Sebastopol, CA 95473
707-824-0914

HOMESPUN FABRICS
PO Box 4315
Thousand Oaks, CA 91359
805-381-0741

J. CREW
1 Ivy Crescent
Lynchburg, VA 24513-1001
800-562-0258

J. JILL
PO Box 3004
Winterbrook Way
Meredith, NH 03253-3004
800-642-9989

JAMIE HARMON
RD 3, Box 464
Jericho, VT 05465
802-879-0800

JANICE CORPORATION
198 Route 46
Budd Lake, NJ 07828
800-526-4237

KIWIS
PO Box 763
Lucerne Valley, CA 92356
619-248-7195

LAND'S END
One Land's End Lane
Dodgeville, WI 53595
800-356-4444

OCARINA TEXTILES
16 Cliff Street
New London, CT 06320
203-437-8189
800-578 4562

THE OHIO HEMPERY
7002 State Route 329
Guysville, OH 45735
800-BUY-HEMP
614-662-4367

ORGANIC COTTONS
103 Hoffecker Road
Phoenixville, PA 19460
610-495-9986

ORGANIC INTERIORS
8 College Avenue
Nanuet, NY 10954
914-623-2114
Fabrics, yarns, and notions

PUEBLO TO PEOPLE
PO Box 2545
Houston, TX 77252-2545
800-843-5257

REFLECTIONS ORGANIC
214 N. Lewis Street
Trinity, TX 75862-9801
800-852-9273
Clothing, footwear.

STRAW INTO GOLD
3006 San Pablo Avenue
Berkeley, CA 94702
510-548-5247
Fabrics, yarns, and notions

SUREWAY TRADING ENTERPRISES
826 Pine Avenue
Niagara Falls, NY 14301-1806
416-596-1887
Fabrics, yarns, and notions

TESTFABRICS
PO Box 420
Middlesex, NJ 08846
908-469-6446
Fabrics, yarns, and notions, kitchen and table linens.

THAI SILKS
252 State Street
Los Altos, CA 94022
800-722-SILK
(in CA: 800-221-SILK)

TWEEDS
One Avery Row
Roanoke, VA 24012-8528
800-999-7997

WINTER SILKS
PO Box 620130
Middleton, WI 53562
800-648-7455

petcare

ALLERGY RESOURCES
PO Box 444
Guffey, CO 80820
800-USE-FLAX

KAREN'S NONTOXIC PRODUCTS
1839 Dr. Jack Road
Conowingo, MD 21918
410-378-4936

NATURAL ANIMAL
7000 US 1 North
St. Augustine, FL 32095
800-274-7387

THE NATURAL PET CARE COMPANY
8050 Lake City Way
Seattle, WA 98115
800-962-8266

SHAMPOO-CHEZ
303 Potrero Street
Building 40-F
Santa Cruz, CA 95060
800-727-PETS

finance

banks & building societies

ENVIRONMENTAL BANKERS ASSOCIATION
110 North Royal St.
Suite 301
Alexandria, VA 22314
703-549-0977
Fax: 1-703-548-5945
envirobank@aol.com
Nonprofit environment bank lender, liability trust, credit, due diligence.

green tourism

ECOSUMMER EXPEDITIONS
PO Box 1765
Clearwater, BC
Canada VOE INO
800-465-8884
www.ecosummer.com

ECO VOYAGER
800-326-7088
www.ecovoyager.com
Specializing in South America

THE INTERNATIONAL ECOTOURISM SOCIETY
PO Box 668
Burlington, VT 05602
802-651-9818
www.ecotourism.org

What to know

This is the "small print" section – the one that gives you additional information on organic principles, regulations, standards, and symbols, so you can shop with confidence and peace of mind.

founding principles

Below are the principles and regulations that underpin organic farming and the production and manufacturing of organic food. The principles of organic agriculture are well defined. No other system of agriculture offers such a complete package of benefits for people or the environment.

AGRICULTURAL PRINCIPLES

❖ Production of high-quality and healthy food in accordance with natural systems.
❖ Respect for natural ecosystems and cycles, from those of the soil to those of plants and animals.
❖ Preservation, maintenance, and increase in the long-term fertility and biological activity of the soil.
❖ Ethical treatment of livestock.
❖ Development of extensive systems based on sustainable production methods.
❖ Respect for traditional practices and recognition of environmental, regional, climatic, and geographic differences.

ENVIRONMENTAL PRINCIPLES

❖ Encouragement of biodiversity and the protection of sensitive habitats and landscape features.
❖ Maximization of renewable resources and recycling.
❖ Minimization of pollution and waste.

FOOD-PROCESSING PRINCIPLES

❖ Minimum processing, consistent with the food product in question.
❖ Restriction of the number of permitted food-processing aids.
❖ Presentation of maximum consumer information on methods of processing and ingredients used.

SOCIAL PRINCIPLES

❖ Provision of fair working conditions and quality of life for workers.
❖ Development of ecologically responsible production, processing, and distribution chains, emphasizing local systems.

STANDARDS FOR ORGANIC FRESH PRODUCE

❖ Generally, a two-year conversion period is required for land before vegetables grown on it can be certified organic, with three years conversion required for orchard fruits and permanent crops such as olives and grapes.
❖ Crops are grown avoiding artificial pesticides and fertilizers.
❖ Pest and diseases are controlled using natural methods, maintaining a diversity of crops and choosing disease-resistant varieties. A small number of permitted sprays, such as soaps, are allowed where necessary.
❖ No post-harvest chemical treatments are allowed, and only natural fruit waxes are allowed.
❖ Crops are grown as part of an integrated mixed cropping system.
❖ Soil fertility is provided by natural fertility-building programs, such as using green manures, supplemented by the use of organic manures and composts and approved organic fertilizers.
❖ Rotation of annual crops is practiced to break pest and disease cycles and to aid and maintain soil fertility and structure.
❖ All genetically modified seeds or other materials that may contain genetically modified organisms (GMOs) are prohibited.

STANDARDS FOR ORGANIC MEAT

Livestock standards are common to all species. Extra standards apply to individual species as appropriate.
❖ Livestock must be born and raised on organic holdings to be sold as organic meat.
❖ Only natural feeds suitable for the species are used, most of which must be organic, although supplementation with limited (specified) amounts of approved nonorganic feeds is allowed when organic is not available.
❖ Animals are allowed to express their natural behavior.
❖ Animals receive no growth promoters, routine veterinary treatments, or antibiotics.
❖ Homeopathy is used widely and, where appropriate, is the preferred method of treatment.
❖ Livestock is raised extensively, not intensively, and is integrated into a diverse farming system.
❖ Animals have continual access to organic grazing pastures or open-air runs as weather permits.
❖ Newborn animals are suckled for as long as possible to enable them to develop natural immunity.

IN ADDITION:

❖ No GMOs are allowed in animal feeds.
❖ Factory farming is banned.
❖ Organophosphate (OP) sheep dips and other OPs to control pests are banned.
❖ There is no teeth-cutting of piglets.
❖ There is no beak-trimming of poultry.
❖ Purchase of animals through livestock markets and export of livestock for slaughter are banned.
❖ Animals bought in as replacement breeding stock or milkers must come with full traceability and from farms with no history of serious diseases; some may come from conventional herds, although their meat cannot be sold as organic at the end of their lives.

additives & processing aids

The following processing aids are considered under organic standards regulations. Each one is under constant review.

ANNATTO   E160(B)

Vegetable dye extracted from the annatto tree. Once widely used to color very pale butter during winter, it is sometimes used to color cheese and other products.

CALCIUM CARBONATE   E170

Natural chalk. Used to reduce excess acidity in wines.

SULPHUR DIOXIDE   E220

Preservative and antioxidant. Allowed only for use in wine and cider to clean out unwanted microbes and to prevent discoloration. Levels allowed are about half to one third those used in conventional production.

SODIUM NITRITE   E250

Derived from sodium nitrate (chile saltpeter). Allowed to be used only in the curing of bacon and ham – it kills the botulinum bacteria and imparts a red color to the meat.

SODIUM NITRATE   E251
POTASSIUM NITRATE   E252

Mined mineral, saltpeter or chile saltpeter. Allowed to be used only in the curing of bacon and ham. Reduces to nitrite, which is the active ingredient in the curing process.

LACTIC ACID   E270

Naturally occurring from lactic bacteria. Used as a food preservative.

CARBON DIOXIDE   E290

Natural gas. Used in carbonated water and soft drinks, also in modified-atmosphere packaging to slow down respiration and to accelerate ripening.

MALIC ACID   E296

Occurs naturally in apples. Used to increase acidity in cider (where low-acidity varieties are used) and in fruit-based foods.

ASCORBIC ACID   E300

Vitamin C. Antioxidant and preservative used in fruit juice; also used as a flour improver.

TOCOPHEROL   E306

Vitamin E (only from natural concentrate, for example wheat germ or soy bean oil). Allowed to be used only as an antioxidant in fats and oils (such as margarine) to prevent them from going rancid.

LECITHINS   E322

Extracted from soy bean oil. Used as an emulsifier in chocolate, margarine, and other foods.

CITRIC ACID   E330
CALCIUM CITRATES   E333

Naturally occurring in citrus fruits. Used as an antioxidant, acidifier, and preservative in fruit products.

TARTARIC ACID   E334
SODIUM TARTRATES   E335

Naturally occurring in grapes. Used as an antioxidant and an acidity regulator.

POTASSIUM TARTRATE   E336

Cream of tartar; used as a raising agent in flour.

MONOCALCIUM PHOSPHATE   E341(A)

Derived from the mineral apatite. Allowed to be used only as a raising agent in self-raising flours.

AGAR   E406

Derived from seaweed. Used as a thickening and gelling agent.

CARRAGEENAN   E407

"Irish Moss," which is derived from seaweed. Used as a stabilizer, thickener, and gelling agent. Only "undegraded" carrageenan is allowed for use, because this is not carcinogenic.

LOCUST BEAN GUM (Carob)   E410
GUAR GUM (Cluster bean)   E412
ARABIC GUM (Acacia)   E414
XANTHAN GUM (fermentation product from corn syrup)   E415

All are extracted from different natural products. They are used as gelling, stabilizing, and thickening agents. Because they each have different properties, they are often used in combination to achieve the specific texture or qualities that are required, for example in sauces, dressings, ice creams, or jellies.

PECTIN   E440(A)

Extracted from fruits. Used as a gelling agent in jams and preserves.

SODIUM CARBONATES   E500
POTASSIUM CARBONATES E501

Bicarbonate of soda. Used as a raising agent in flour and in the processing of sugar.

AMMONIUM CARBONATES   E503

Made by mixing chalk and ammonium sulphate. Used as a raising agent in flour and baked products.

CALCIUM CHLORIDE   E509

Derived from natural salt brines. Allowed to be used only as a coagulation agent, for example in tofu.

CALCIUM SULPHATE   E516

Gypsum. Allowed only as a carrier, for example for the minerals and vitamins that are required by law in white flour, or as a coagulation agent, for example in tofu.

SODIUM HYDROXIDE   E524

Caustic soda. Allowed only in "Hugengebäck" (a traditional German pastry), in the processing of beet sugar, and as an oxidizing agent for black olives.

NITROGEN   E931
OXYGEN   E948

Natural gases. Used in modified-atmosphere packaging.

SODIUM CHLORIDE or POTASSIUM CHLORIDE

Natural salt. Used widely as a flavor enhancer and preservative. A flowing agent may be used where it can be proved to be necessary, to ensure even application in the manufacturing process.

MAGNESIUM CHLORIDE

Otherwise known as nigari. Allowed to be used only as a coagulation agent, for example for tofu.

standards count

Organic farmers are the only farmers whose working practices and standards are enshrined by law and are so strictly policed and enforced. Every farmer, producer, processor, or manufacturer of organic foods and other goods must be certified by a recognized body. They have to undergo a rigorous annual inspection and must keep full records of every transaction and all working practices. In this way, full traceability from farm to table is guaranteed. Enforcing and maintaining standards is a costly but necessary business. It is important for consumer confidence and for the integrity of the organic movement. Standards provide farmers with a manual of how to farm organically. They also provide processors and manufacturers with rules about how to process their products and avoid any potential contamination with conventional produce. The rules cover everything from the time the seed is first planted to how the food is packaged. Standards are also at the cutting edge of organic farming and, as it evolves and organic food becomes mainstream, they are constantly being refined and improved to reflect this evolutionary process. The basic tenets and practices, however, remain steadfast: a partnership with nature for the production of healthy food through healthy soil, the protection of biodiversity and the environment, and sustainable farming solutions that will benefit us all for the future.

reading the labels

All the information you need to know about an organic product can be found on the label:

✤ **The word "organic"** – only goods that have been independently certified as organic can use this word in their title.

✤ **Certification logo & number** – the consumer guarantee that a product is genuinely organic.

✤ **Ingredients list** – all organic ingredients are clearly marked; any permitted nonorganic ingredients will also be listed.

✤ **Food you can trust** – organic products often carry information about what organic farming is, or more about the producer.

ORGANIC FOODS

✤ If the word "organic" appears in the title, as in "Organic Baked Beans," this means that the contents must be composed of a mandated minimum of products organic in origin, but up to a small percent may also be from a short list of permitted nonorganic ingredients.

✤ If the title says "Baked Beans with 70, 80, or 90 percent organic ingredients," for example, it means that the stated percentage is of organic contents; the rest is from the shortlist of permitted nonorganic ingredients.

OTHER PRODUCTS

Organic certification covers chiefly food and primary agricultural products. In addition, organic standards for nonfood products, such as clothing, are certified by a number of certifying bodies. The overall status of organic certification is constantly changing as consumer demand for organic products increases and regulatory bodies are created to oversee all aspects of organic production.

a rough guide to standards

The US is still working toward nationally agreed organic standards, as is Japan. The UK, on the other hand, has five officially recognized certification bodies, whose symbols or certification numbers you will find on the foods they have certified. Each certification agency in the UK is an organization its own right, with its own set of standards and members who pay a fee every year for its services, including an annual inspection. Each agency's standards must, at the very least, conform to the official standards laid down by the overall governing body, the UK Register of Organic Food Standards (UKROFS), which in turn conform to the organic regulations laid down by the European Union (EU). UKROFS is an independent body, designated by the Ministry of Agriculture, which sets and maintains organic standards in the UK and administers EU organic regulations.

At a global level these standards are themselves influenced by the Codex Alimentarius (an international committee on food labeling) and by the International Federation of Organic Agricultural Movements (IFOAM), an independent organization that has over 700 member organizations in more than 100 countries. Being interrelated this way provides the structure for eventual harmonization of organic standards.

Worldwide there are several hundred certifying bodies. Any products that are imported into the EU must have equivalent certification standards to those in the EU, and be approved by an EU certifying body, again ensuring basic harmonization. Most certifying bodies are also members of IFOAM. This organization has its own accrediting body, IFOAM Accreditation (International Organic Accreditation Services Inc.), that approves and accredits those organizations that meet its own high international standards. Currently 15 different certification organizations have been accredited by IFOAM Accreditation, and all are bound by IFOAM's standards. The result is a simpler certification process for farmers wanting to export crops, and reassurance for the consumer that imported crops certified by IFOAM-accredited organizations have been produced to the same high standards worldwide.

KNOW YOUR ORGANIC RIGHTS

It is important for everyone that organic standards are upheld at all times. Use this simple guide to help the organic movement police standards by checking products when you shop.
♣ Only food certified as organic can legally be sold as organic, so be sure to look for a certification symbol or number alongside the word "organic."
♣ Organic producers and manufacturers must be able to provide proof of authenticity if required, so do not hesitate to ask if you want to check where something came from.
♣ It is usually unacceptable for any retailer to repackage organic goods out of sight of the customer (including local home deliveries), unless the store itself has also been certified by a recognized organic certification body.
♣ All manufacturers and processors producing foods that are labeled organic should be registered with an organic certification body themselves.

Index

C

cabbages 59
cakes, cookies, & candies 94, 95
Camphill Communities 80, 223
Canada, apples, & pears 65
Canary Islands, tomatoes 53
carrots 27, 52, 58
caterpillars 163
cats, feeding, & care 210, 212–13
cattle 18, 19, 41, 76
cauliflower 54
celeriac 58
celery 58
centipedes 150, 159
Centre for Alternative Technology
   181, 197, 217, 226
cereals & grains
   for animals 210–11
   breakfast 72, 76
   see also individually by name
     e.g. wheat
certification
   see standards & certification
chaffs 211
chamomile tea 105, 133
chard 59, 171
Charles, Prince of Wales 30, 40–1
cheese 71, 80
chemicals
   conventional farming use 20
   see also by type e.g. pesticides
cherries 175
chervil 171
chicken 86, 87, 88
chicory 61, 170
Chile, fruit 65, 66
chilled & frozen foods 98–9
China 33
   factory farming 29
   hemp 202
   silk 203
   soil erosion 17
Chinese leaves 60
chocolate 95
chutneys & preserves 94
ciders 109
cilantro 171

citrus fruits 66
Clark, Nikki 141
clay soils 151
cleaning products 184–5
   addresses & websites 241
climbing plants for the garden 149
clothes *see* fabrics, fibers & clothes
clove oil 133
clover 154
clubroot 163
Co-operative Bank 217
cooperatives
   consumer 38
   in developing world 95, 221
   finance 218
   milk producers 41, 77, 81
coffee & tea 35, 104–5
   addresses & websites 236
cognac & brandies 108
colas 106
cold-pressed oils 89
colors, artificial, in cosmetics, 140
comfrey liquid 155
community farms & gardens 38–9
complementary therapies 132–3
   for pets 207, 212
composite boards 193
compost
   garden compost 152–3
   local authority/community
     compost 155, 226
   production & use in vineyards
     112, 113
   recycling organic waste 182
computer equipment 189
conservation, on organic farms
   19, 22–3
consumer cooperatives 38
consumerism 219
container gardening 149, 168,
   171, 174
containers, compost 152
conventional farming
   aims & principles 15
   biodiversity & conservation 18,
     20, 22, 41
   chemical use 20, 24–5
   crop health 26–7
   economics, yields &
     profitability 41, 43, 83

genetically modified organisms
   (GMOs) 30–1
   livestock farming 28–9
   soil quality 17
conversion period & derogation,
   organic farming 43, 51
Cook Islands, organic farming 33
cookies, cakes, & candies 94, 95
corn 56–7
cosmetics
   see beauty products, cosmetics
     & toiletries
cot mattresses 125
cotton & cotton products 202,
   204–5
   baby clothes 124–5
   home furnishings, & linens 188
cranberries 36, 64
Cranberry Hill Organic Farm 36
credit cards 217
credit unions 216, 243
cress 170
crimson clover 154
crops
   crop health & harmony
     research 26–7
   diversity on organic farms 19
   genetically modified (GM)
     30–1, 56–7, 100
   rotations 20, 51
   see also individual crops by
     name e.g. soy beans
crystalization techniques 26–7
cupboard & pantry products 90, 91
Cuba, organic farming 32
currencies, alternative 216

d

dairies & dairy products 80–1
   addresses & websites 236
   see also individual dairy
     products by name e.g. cheese
dark green vegetables 59
dates 67
detoxification 132

dehydration 131
delicatessen products 78, 98–9
Demeter label 43, 209
Denmark 32
   crop health & harmony
     research 26
derogation & conversion period,
   organic farming 43, 51
derris 162, 163
design
   see planning & design
detergents & cleaning products
   184–5
   addresses & websites 241
devil's claw 63
diapers 122-24
diapers & baby wipes 122-3
diaper rash 124
address & websites 237
Dick, Jane 121
dill 171
dinner 84–5
directories, books & magazines
   228–31
disease control
   see pest & disease control
disposable diapers 122–4
DIY products
   addresses & websites 239–41
   composite boards & fixings 193
   insulation 193
   paints, stains & varnishes 192–3
   timber & wood-based products
     180, 187, 190–1
dogs, feeding, & care 209–10,
   212–13
Dominican Republic, bananas 68,
   69
Dr. Hauschka beauty products 137
dressings & sauces 93, 94, 100,
   101
drinks 103 *see also* individually by
name, e.g. wine
drugs & medicines 129, 130
dry-cleaning 199
D'Silva, Joyce 29
Duchy Home Farm, Highgrove
   40–1
Duchy Originals 41
ducks 35–6

l

m

n

o

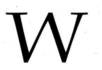
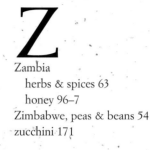

Acknowledgments

AUTHOR'S ACKNOWLEDGMENTS

This book is organic in content and organic by nature, and would never have been possible without the cooperation and goodwill of the many people who have worked so hard, or who have given their help so generously, to make this book so special. The credit for the book belongs entirely to them and I should like to acknowledge my profound gratitude and respect to everyone involved.

First and foremost, for giving their best, and for enriching the book in so many ways, I should like to express my particular thanks to my fellow contributors and to everyone who has kindly provided quotes for us. For use of their work and their help, I should also like to offer my sincere thanks to Dr. Ursula Balzer-Graf, Dr. Louise Drinkwater, Thomas B. Harding, Dr. Mae-wan Ho, Dr. Harald Hoppe, Professor Angelika Meier-Ploeger, Dr. Urs Niggli, Jens-Otto Anderson, Professor David Pimentel, and Dr. Bodil Søgaard.

An author's role is to produce words, but it is the design and editorial team that makes a book come alive. For working like heroes under impossible circumstances and even more impossible deadlines, and producing dazzling results, my thanks to all at Dorling Kindersley. In particular, I owe a profound debt of gratitude to David Summers and to my editor, Stephanie Farrow, for their unfailing consideration, professionalism, and kindness throughout. For Stephanie, for having abundant good grace, and the patience of an angel that I didn't deserve, and for helping us all achieve the impossible, I should like to express my deep respect and fondest affection.

Organics brings out the best in people. For their generosity and personal support, my heartfelt thanks to Howard-Yana Shapiro and Anthony Rodale. For being an unpaid knight in shining armor, my especial thanks to Peter Segger.

I should also like to acknowledge and thank the many manufacturers and producers, fair trade, economic, and GM experts and others I have consulted. These include: Lawrence Woodward, Paul Burgess, Iain Tolehurst, Robert Duxbury, Allan Kay, Jim Freimuth, Matthew Wilson, Ian Pardoe, Pam Seldon, Robert Crone, Peter Hall, John Richards, Malcolm Hensby, Alex Pearce, Nancy Evans, Kristine Kreese, Gaye and Mike Donaldson, Cyril Lombard, Sally Bagenall, Clare Marriage, Nigel Woodhouse, Robert Wilson, Lorraine Brehme, Mark Woollard, Chris Dawson, John Belleme, Liz Parker, Alistair Smith, Judith Houston, Phil Wells, Alistair Menzies, Anna Chipchase, Jess Day, Dr. Götz E. Rehn, Susan Jenkins, Simon Roberts, Lee V. Coates, Sue Mayer, Sue Dibb, Leonie Green, Lindsay Keegan, George Smith, Tania Maxted-Frost, Bjarne Pedersen, Karen Witt Olsen, Claire Jackson, Simon Wright, Craig Sams, Neil Palmer, Bob Lloyd, and Michelle Berriedale-Johnson.

The Soil Association has been immensely helpful. Here I should like to pay particular tribute to Francis Blake and Rob Haward, both of whom gave invaluable guidance; also to Patrick Holden, Phil Stocker, Martin Trowell, Philip Prideux, Emma Parkin, Dom Lane, and the staff of the Local Food Links Team. I should also like to thank the staff at Friends of the Earth, especially Adrian Bebb and Sandra Bell, Jim Thomas at Greenpeace, and Mark Griffiths of the Natural Law Party.

For their diligent research work, their support, and for never squawking, many thanks to Jan Deane and Rachel Vosper; and also to Louise Cairns for being the most helpful and efficient PR in the business.

On a personal front, warm and many affectionate thanks to Rosie for giving me wings and letting me fly; to my agent, Rosemary Scoular at PFD, for listening endlessly and for always being cheerful; to Angela Mason at *YOU Magazine*, for her support and for teaching me more than she could ever guess; and, for working magic, the House of Good Health in Henley-on-Thames and Sigyta Hart.

I wish there was an easy way to write a book. For being there in so many different ways, for Joanna, my lifelong thanks. For bearing the brunt, for Rick, my love. I promise to try and do better next time.

PUBLISHER'S ACKNOWLEDGMENTS

Dorling Kindersley would like to thank Neil Lockley and Mark Wallace for editorial work and Sue Costen, Ros Saunders, Poppy Jenkins, and Sara Williams for design assistance. Thanks to Sue Bosanko for compiling the index, and to Anna Grapes and Claire Gouldstone for picture research.

For his stunning photography thanks to Ian O'Leary. Many thanks also for their invaluable help and support to Howard-Yana Shapiro, Anthony Rodale and Peter Segger. For assistance with sourcing images and props for photography thanks to Scott Vlaun, Todd Greb, Green Baby, Texture, Dr. Mae-wan Ho, Karl Ludwig Schweisfurth and the Herrmannsdorfer Landwerkstätten, Sheepdrove Farm, Sally Fox, Diane Godwin at the National Federation of City Farms, Clopton Flowers, Vicky Pollitt, Hilary Cook, Liz and Bob Farrow, Green People, Gerd Weiss, Binnie Brown, Cranberry Hill Farm, Jim Freimuth, Monika Kilb and the Sekem cotton initiative, Jason Griffiths, Pascoe's, Auro Paints, Casa Paints, Aveda, Jurlique, Neal's Yard, Cariad Aromatherapy, Origins, Dr. Hauschka, Lu Setnicka and Isabelle Moreau of Patagonia, and Rocombe Farm. Thanks too to the Aldeburgh Festival for help in sourcing the pictures on pages 82–83.